The Management of the Diabetic Foot

To Rosemary and Anne, Katherine,
Christopher and David

For Churchill Livingstone
Publisher: Peter Richardson
Editorial Co-ordination: Editorial Resources Unit
Production Controller: Neil Dickson
Design: Design Resources Unit
Sales Promotion Executive: Louise Johnstone

The Management of the Diabetic Foot

Irwin Faris MB BS (Melb) MD (Monash) FRACS
Chairman, Department of Surgery, University of Adelaide;
Head of Unit of Vascular Surgery, Royal Adelaide Hospital.
Formerly John Astor Fellow, The Middlesex Hospital Medical School;
Wellcome Clinical Research Fellow, Royal Postgraduate Medical School,
London.

With contributions from
Pamela M. Le Quesne DM FRCP and
Nicholas Parkhouse DM FRCS
Department of Neurological Studies,
University College and Middlesex School of Medicine,
London

SECOND EDITION

CHURCHILL LIVINGSTONE
EDINBURGH LONDON MELBOURNE NEW YORK AND TOKYO 1991

CHURCHILL LIVINGSTONE
Medical Division of Longman Group UK Limited

Distributed in the United States of America by Churchill
Livingstone Inc., 1560 Broadway, New York, N.Y. 10036, and
by associated companies, branches and representatives
throughout the world.

ISBN 0-443-04249-7

First edition 1982
Second edition 1991

British Library Cataloguing in Publication Data
CIP Catalogue record for this book is available from
the British Library
Library of Congress Cataloging in Publication Data
CIP Catalog record for this book is available from
the Library of Congress

Produced by Longman Singapore Publishers Pte Ltd
Printed in Singapore

Preface

In the nine years since the preparation of the first edition of this book there have been a number of areas in which we have increased our understanding of the processes which underly the development of foot lesions in diabetic patients. These include new knowledge relating to the function of small blood vessels which has improved our understanding of the possible mechanisms for the development of microangiopathy and an improved understanding of the metabolic functions in the peripheral nerve fibres which has helped our understanding of the development of peripheral neuropathy. However in neither case do we yet have a complete understanding of the processes nor do we have effective means of preventing the development of the complications of diabetes. There has been a greatly increased understanding of the pathophysiology of microvascular and autonomic nervous function and this has helped us define more clearly the disturbances which are present. Most important of all is the clinical experience gathered in the intervening years which has caused a development of ideas relating to the optimum means of treatment. All these reasons justify revision of the original text.

My original aim was to provide a concise account of the processes involved in the development of foot lesions 'at a level which can be understood by anyone concerned in the care of these patients.' A number of colleagues from different disciplines in different countries have been kind enough to say that they have found the first edition a help in the management of their patients. This has been very gratifying to me and I hope that this revision will continue to fulfil those expectations.

All sections of the book have been revised and many rewritten. I am most grateful for the collaboration of Dr Pamela Le Quesne and Mr Nicholas Parkhouse who have rewritten the chapter on Neuropathy which is now well outside my area of expertise. I am sure that this chapter is much improved. Dr Ross Smith, Clinical Microbiologist at the Institute of Medical and Veterinary Science, Adelaide made helpful suggestions about the sections on microbiology and antibiotic therapy. Finally I am grateful to my colleagues in the Vascular Surgery Unit at the Royal Adelaide Hospital for their continued support and encouragement in the many discussions we have had during ward rounds about the management of individual patients.

Adelaide, 1991   I. F.

Foreword to the First Edition

Notwithstanding the fact that the fundamental defect affects carbohydrate metabolism, diabetes mellitus is a disease with widespread effects throughout the body, and the care of the diabetic patient may well comprise a multiplicity of problems, involving many organs and systems, notably the eyes, the kidneys, the blood vessels and the peripheral nerves. It is likely that with improved control of the underlying metabolic defect — a goal that seems within reach with various techniques currently under investigation — the incidence of these complications of diabetes mellitus will fall, and there can be no question that in the long term the goal to be achieved is their prevention rather than their management. None the less, at the present time it remains the case that these complications are an important cause of disability and real distress for many patients with this common disease, and their management constitutes an essential part of the care of many diabetics.

An important group amongst diabetic patients presenting problems due to these complications is formed by those with problems affecting the foot. Although not as common as some other complications, such as those affecting the eye, these are of particular importance to the patient as ultimately they may lead to the necessity for amputation of the foot or lower leg. This will result in grave disability if, as is tragically only too often the case, the patient's eyesight is also impaired. This group is also of great importance to the Health Services because of the long periods of hospital care that these patients may require. The foot complications are due to a variety of causes, notably arterial disease, peripheral neuropathy and skeletal deformity, often with sepsis complicating the picture. Probably because of this multiplicity of causative factors, their complications have tended to fall into a no-man's land between orthopaedic, vascular and general surgeons, diabetic physicians and chiropodists. As a result, they have not, in general, received the expert, detailed study they merit.

However, in recent years growing attention has been paid to the causes and management of the foot problems that beset diabetic patients, and the time is ripe for a book such as this to bring together our increasing understanding of this inter-related group of conditions. With a long-standing interest in these problems Mr Faris has himself carried out important studies into various aspects of the neuropathic complications. Furthermore, he is an experienced vascular surgeon. He is thus ideally equipped by the pattern of his clinical experience and by his combination of clinical and research expertise in the field, to master the interlocking factors that contribute to the totality of the 'diabetic foot'. In this admirably lucid book Mr Faris surveys the whole field related to our understanding and management of these problems. By bringing together in this single volume all the different aspects of problems which, although anatomically circumscribed in their clinical manifestations, are wide-ranging in the physiological and pathological disturbances involved, Mr Faris enables the whole problem of the 'diabetic foot' to be seen and comprehended in its entirety. As such this book is a much-needed addition to the bibliography of diabetes mellitus.

I have for many years been involved in the care of diabetic patients with foot problems, and for some time have felt that a book of this scope was needed. It is, therefore, a real privilege to be asked to write this foreword to this admirable book, which should help many clinicians, both physicians and surgeons, to a clearer understanding of these difficult problems, and thus help many patients to whom these complications of diabetes can be a great burden.

1982   L. P. Le Quesne

Contents

1. A brief history of diabetes and its complications

Diabetes is one of many common diseases known from antiquity. A disease with polyuria is mentioned in the Ebers papyrus which includes Egyptian medical compilations dating from the second millenium B.C. In the middle of the second Christian century Aretaeus of Cappodocia used the Greek word for a syphon δ ιαβητηζ to describe a disease in which water did not remain long in the body. The features included thirst, weight loss and polyuria. At about the same time Galen attributed this disease to the inability of the kidneys to retain water so that it passed through unchanged. The first account of sweet urine was reportedly given in India about 500 A.D. This preceded by more than 1000 years the account of Thomas Willis in 1675. In addition, it was recognized that there was a less harmful form of the disease in which the urine was tasteless.

In the second half of the eighteenth century, important advances were made. Robert Wyatt found a sugar-like substance in urine following evaporation. In the same period Frank classified the disease into two forms: diabetes insipidus (or spurious) in which there was no sugar in the urine, or diabetes mellitus (or vera) in which the urine contained sugar.

The modern era can be said to have begun with the work of John Rollo who in 1798 concluded that diabetes was a disease of the stomach which resulted in the abnormal transformation of vegetable nutritive matter into sugar. He prescribed a treatment regimen of carbohydrate restriction which soon fell from favour because it might well have been worse than the disease. In the nineteenth century, progress was rapid. McGregor and Magendie separately found sugar both in the blood of diabetics and, in small quantities, in blood from normal subjects. More detailed knowledge of the metabolism of sugar had to await the studies of Claude Bernard.

Early suggestions that the pancreas was involved in diabetes followed the 1885 observation that administration of phloridzin to an animal was followed by glycosuria. The classic experiments of pancreatic ablation were performed shortly afterwards by Von Mering and Minkowski although they had been attempted 40 years earlier by Bouchardat. The link between the pancreas and diabetes was unknown but the disease could be prevented by transplanting a fragment of the pancreas. In 1892 Lepine proposed that

1

diabetes was due to the absence of a glycolytic ferment in the pancreatic juice but pathological confirmation of the link was not achieved until Opie in 1900 demonstrated the connection between disease of the islets of Langerhans and diabetes. Sharpey-Schafer concluded that the islands of Langerhans must secrete a substance which regulated carbohydrate metabolism, and in 1916, proposed the name of insulin for this hypothetical substance.

The discovery of insulin in 1921 ranks with the discovery of penicillin and streptomycin in the benefit it conferred to sufferers of an incurable lethal disease. Bliss (1988) described the impact of the discovery thus:

Those who watched the first starved, sometimes comatose, diabetics receive insulin and return to life saw one of the genuine miracles of modern medicine. They were present at the closest approach to the resurrection of the body that our secular society can achieve.

Bliss's book provides an historian's view of the events in Toronto in 1921–1923 and is fascinating reading for anyone with an interest in the care of diabetic patients. The book by Wrenshall (1962) also gives a vivid account of this dramatic period though it does not attempt to give the same detail.

Following the introduction of insulin, when death in coma became a less frequent outcome of the disease, attention began to be turned to the longer-term complications and it was soon recognized that deaths from vascular disease had become more common.

John Rollo (1798) first recognized an association between diabetes and symptoms in the limbs. His patient had pains and paraesthesiae: 'lumbago and sciatica in so great a degree as to be nearly deprived of the use of the lower limbs'. Indeed before 1850 the frequency of neurological changes in diabetics led to suggestions that neuropathy was the cause of diabetes. Between 1850 and 1870 both gangrene and plantar ulcers were recognized as complications of diabetes. In 1888 Hunt collected 72 cases of diabetic gangrene and concluded that 'gangrene in diabetes is something more than a coincidence'. During the last 30 years of the century there were rapid advances in understanding of neurological complications. Absence of tendon reflexes, abnormalities of sweating and motor paralysis were described and pathological examination revealed degenerative changes in the peripheral nerve and the dorsal columns of the spinal cord.

The association between foot ulceration, neuropathy and vascular disease was first recorded by Pryce (1887):

The patient was a 56-year-old man who had symptoms of diabetes for 18 months. For 3 months he had noticed ulceration on the regions of the first right metatarsophalangeal joint and the fifth left metatarsophalangeal joint. There was decreased sensation of the lower one third of the legs and feet and the knee jerks were absent. The legs were livid and cold. Death in coma occurred 4 days later. At autopsy degenerative changes were noted in the dorsal and lumbar parts of the spinal cord and in the peripheral nerves. There was atheromatous disease of the posterior tibial arteries and of its smallest branches.

In 1893 he reported two further cases. In each case there was marked atheroma of the posterior tibial artery and 'blocking up of smaller microscopic blood vessels'. His conclusions were, that while neuritis in young diabetics might be due to a specific toxic poison, in older subjects it was due to vascular disease. The idea that vascular disease was the cause of neuritis, ulceration and gangrene was for the next 50 years the dominant influence both on thoughts on the pathogenesis of foot lesions and in plans of treatment.

The emphasis on vascular disease as a cause of foot lesions meant that until quite recently major amputations were performed frequently, sometimes for small areas of gangrene. In the pre-antibiotic era the mortality in these patients was very high and many patients were treated by their physicians for long periods, perhaps because they feared that major amputation was the only alternative. Some surgeons were able to report occasional successes with local amputation but clear indications for local or major amputation were not established for much of this period. Thus the success of local treatment in selected cases had been demonstrated but it is clear that these were the fortunate patients; inability to control the diabetes and spreading sepsis caused the death of many.

In the period 1920–1950 arterial disease was believed to be the dominant factor in the development of foot lesions. The hypothesis that disease of the microscopic blood vessels might be the cause of several of the major complications of diabetes was put forward in 1941 when the association between retinopathy, neuropathy and nephropathy was noted and the suggestion made that the common factor was disease of the blood vessels. This view was reinforced by reports in 1959 in which changes in the vessels in amputated limbs and in small nerve biopsies were described (see Ch 4). However, observations of a dissociation between vascular disease and neuropathy gave rise to two important changes in opinion:

1. Metabolic rather than vascular factors might cause neuropathy
2. Neuropathy, independent of vascular disease, might cause foot lesions.

This latter view was most clearly recognised by Oakley et al who in 1956 described the classification of foot lesions which provides the basis for most contemporary classifications.

Since the 1950s the techniques of arterial reconstruction have been applied increasingly to the management of these patients. These techniques have developed to the extent that bypass grafts can be attached to the arteries of the ankle or foot, thus avoiding amputation in a number of patients. In the past 10 years there has been a re-awakening of interest in the pathophysiology of vascular disease in the diabetic limb. This has been aided by the development of new methods for the study of the circulation in the limbs. As a result we are now in a position to understand more clearly the role of the various aetiological factors and thus plan treatment more rationally than before.

REFERENCES

Bliss M 1988 The discovery of insulin. Faber and Faber, London
Oakley W, Catterall R C F, Martin M M 1956 Aetiology and management of lesions of the
    feet in diabetics. British Medical Journal 2: 953–957
Pryce T D 1887 A case of perforating ulcers of both feet with diabetes and ataxic
    symptoms. Lancet 2: 11–12
Rollo J 1798 Cases of the diabetes mellitus, 2nd edn. C Dilly, London, p 260
Wrenshall G A, Hetenyi G, Feasby W R, Marcus A 1962 The story of insulin. The Bodley
    Head, London

2. Mechanisms for the development of foot lesions

The classification of Oakley et al (1956) was a major contribution to our understanding of the causes of foot problems in diabetic patients. They classified the causes as: (1) ischaemia, (2) neuropathy, (3) infection, (4) combined. This outline is the basis of current classifications which have been presented in a more detailed form (see Du Plessis 1970).

The complications of diabetes predispose to the development of foot lesions. These complications are largely irreversible and the onset is unpredictable. When they occur the foot becomes vulnerable, yet patients may live for many years and eventually die from another manifestation of the vascular disease, e.g. nephropathy or myocardial infarction, without ever having a significant foot infection or ulcer. This is because these patients have avoided the precipitating factors, of which the most important is mechanical trauma. Minor wounds or infections in a foot with normal sensation and normal blood supply are recognized by the pain they cause so they are treated early and heal rapidly. In the anaesthetic foot a small lesion may progress because it is not recognized and the source of injury not removed. Impairment of the blood supply may result in delayed healing. Infection is an important aggravating factor which may cause extensive tissue damage.

In this chapter an outline of the pathogenic mechanisms will be given. Detailed discussion of their occurrence and importance is given in subsequent chapters. The factors responsible for the development of foot problems in diabetics (see Fig. 2.1) can be classified as:

Predisposing Factors
    Vascular disease
    Neuropathy
    Liability to infection
Precipitating Factors
    Physical injury, i.e.
    Mechanical trauma
    Heat
Aggravating factors
    Infection
    Ischaemia
    Neuropathy.

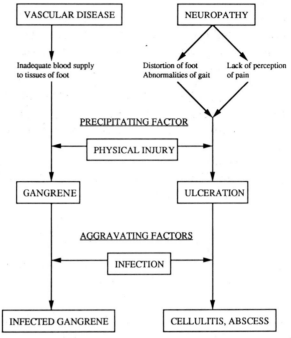

Fig. 2.1   Predisposing, precipitating and aggravating factors and some of their interactions.

PREDISPOSING FACTORS

Vascular disease (Ch. 3)

Atherosclerosis.   This may cause ischaemic foot lesions in diabetics just as it does in non-diabetics, and is the most important factor in about half the patients seen in developed countries. If the blood supply to the foot is reduced sufficiently, minor wounds will not heal and there may be ischaemic pain at rest. Neuropathy frequently coexists and is a mixed blessing: the patient is spared the pain of an ischaemic foot, but tissue damage and infection may progress unnoticed.

Calcification of arteries.   This is an indicator of a prolonged diabetic metabolic disturbance but there is no evidence that it is an important factor in the development of foot problems.

Microangiopathy.   The role of disease of arterioles and capillaries is still controversial. If the disease were sufficiently widespread, local blood flow might be reduced to such a degree that ischaemic lesions could develop and extend as outlined above, and the rigidity of the vessel walls might reduce the ability of the microcirculation to respond to injury and mount an adequate inflammatory response. The role of microangiopathy is discussed on page 36.

Neuropathy (Ch. 4)

The major components are:

Loss of perception of pain. This and ischaemia are the two most important factors in the development of severe foot lesions. Impaired perception of pain means that small injuries go unrecognized and thus progress before diagnosis. This often causes loss of tissue, but there is no direct evidence that neuropathy aids the development of infection.

Paralysis of the small muscles of the foot. This results in clawing of the toes and a decreased effective load-bearing area under the forefoot. Thus abnormal forces may affect both the deformed toes and the area of the metatarsal heads.

Autonomic neuropathy. This might potentiate the development of lesions by (1) failure of reflex dilatation in response to local injury; (2) abnormal vasoconstriction in response to cold (see p 51).

PRECIPITATING FACTORS

Despite the presence of predisposing factors an uninjured foot may not develop serious problems. However physical trauma is a potent cause of trouble (see Ch. 6).

1. A puncture wound, e.g. from ingrowing toenail, will allow the entry of bacteria and infection may result. In addition, if there is severe ischaemia of the tissues, progressive necrosis may follow.

2. Localized pressure, e.g. from tight shoes, may cause ischaemic necrosis.

3. Repeated mechanical trauma, e.g. from walking, may cause inflammation and subsequent necrosis.

4. Heat, e.g. from a hot water bottle, may burn the skin if there is reduced perception of temperature and pain sensation.

In addition, chemical injury may result from the application of corrosive substances, e.g. in corn plasters.

AGGRAVATING FACTORS

Infection (Ch. 5)

This is an important factor responsible for increasing the amount of damaged tissue. As a result of infection a limb may be lost despite the presence of an adequate blood supply. Decreased resistance will accentuate the effect of infection but in almost every case bacteria gain access to the tissues following mechanical trauma. The possible mechanisms are discussed in Chapter 5 and include:

1. Abnormal cellular and humoral responses to inflammation. This

may be potentiated by impairment of the blood supply and, perhaps, dysfunction of the autonomic nervous system.

2. Decreased efficiency of the process of repair, the most important component of which is collagen formation.

Ischaemia

This also acts as an aggravating factor:

1. Because healing of minor lesions is impaired as a result of the inability to increase the local blood supply. This deficit may also predispose to the spread of infection;

2. By providing an environment which allows the growth of anaerobic bacteria.

Neuropathy

Loss of pain sensation acts as an aggravating factor by permitting mechanical injury and infection to continue unnoticed.

This concept of predisposing, precipitating and aggravating factors has important implications for the management of diabetic patients who may have vascular disease and/or neuropathy but will not develop lesions unless exposed to a precipitating factor. Even at this stage, resolution of the problem can be expected if the effects of the potential aggravating factor can be avoided (e.g. by aggressive treatment of minor infection or by removing sources of mechanical trauma). In general the vascular disease and neuropathy cannot be reversed (although their development may be delayed). However the precipitating factors may be regarded as preventable and thus the rigorous avoidance of physical trauma would prevent the development of most of these problems which occupy so much of the resources of our hospitals and clinics. This preventative approach is emphasized in Chapter 7. Unfortunately these tactics often fail and Chapters 9 and 10 describes the methods of assessment and treatment for the salvage of these limbs.

REFERENCES

Oakley W, Caterall R C F, Martin M M 1956 Aetiology and management of lesions of the feet in diabetics. British Medical Journal 2: 953–957
Du Plessis D J 1970 Lesions on the feet in patients with diabetes mellitus. South African Journal of Surgery 8: 29–46

3. Vascular disease

INTRODUCTION

Disease of blood vessels is a major cause of complications in diabetics. It may affect both capillaries, the smallest blood vessels across which nutrient exchange occurs in the tissues, and the largest arteries, the aorta and its branches. Obstruction of the larger vessels may cause the complications of stroke or myocardial infarction while disease of the smaller vessels causes loss of vision (diabetes is the commonest cause of blindness in many Western communities) and kidney failure. The following sections give accounts of the types of arterial disease, their prevalence and aetiology.

Earlier descriptions of vascular disease relied on the morbid anatomical appearances of arteries and histological sections of various tissues. In recent years a wide variety of methods have been used for studying the circulation in the living limb. These methods have given a much more detailed, but still incomplete account of the changes that occur. As a consequence, our understanding of aetiology and mechanisms of production of disease has expanded rapidly.

Disease is commonly described as affecting large or small vessels. The unqualified use of the term 'small vessel disease' has often made understanding of this subject very difficult, particularly when considering possible effects on the foot. The term may be given several meanings:

1. Disease of arterioles and capillaries (i.e. synonymous with 'microangiopathy'). Small vessel disease in this context has often been inappropriately blamed as a cause of foot changes that were primarily due to neuropathy. The situation has been clarified in recent years and will be discussed in this chapter.

2. Disease of arteries in the calf. To vascular surgeons these are 'small vessels', disease of which may lead to amputation because of the lack of a suitable vessel to receive a bypass graft. However, bypass grafting is now being performed regularly to vessels at the level of the ankle joint.

3. The metatarsal and digital arteries are also affected by disease which resembles atherosclerosis, although its importance is uncertain.

The term 'small vessel disease' must be used carefully so that the sorts of vessels being considered are defined clearly.

9

The elements of the peripheral circulation are:

1. Arteries which carry the blood from the heart to the periphery.
2. Microcirculation, which includes small arteries and arterioles whose function is concerned with the regulation of peripheral resistance and hence arterial blood pressure; capillaries across which nutrient exchange takes place; and venules which collect the blood which has passed through the capillaries. In certain areas of the body there are arteriovenous communications which, when open, allow the blood to bypass the capillary bed.
3. Veins which return blood to the heart.
4. Lymphatics which collect protein, macromolecules and excess fluid which cannot re-enter the capillaries and return these materials to the circulation.

Table 3.1 shows these components plus other elements involved in the regulation of the peripheral circulation and indicates that diabetes causes a disturbance in almost all of them. This chapter discusses the aetiology, occurrence and effects of these disorders in diabetic patients, particularly as they affect the circulation to the lower limb.

ATHEROSCLEROSIS

Atherosclerosis is the commonest cause of death in many Western societies. It may be defined as a degenerative vascular disease, composed of fibrous and/or fatty change affecting principally the tunica intima of arteries. Ulceration and secondary thrombosis commonly occur. It has been believed for many years that this condition occurs more frequently and with greater severity in diabetics and the epidemiological evidence to support this view is now very strong (see West 1978). There are several lines of evidence which support the view that there is an increased occurrence of vascular disease in diabetics.

Community surveys

The best evidence has come from prospective studies involving large samples of patients from single communities. These studies have been carried out in many regions — North America, Scandinavia, eastern Europe, South Africa, Great Britain, Australia — with similar results. They show that both the prevalence and the incidence of vascular disease is increased in diabetics. The study carried out in Framingham, Massachusetts, demonstrated that diabetes was an independent risk factor in the development of coronary heart disease. The incidence of cardiovascular disease (coronary, cerebral and peripheral) was increased, and the risk of death from cardiovascular disease was increased more in women than in men (Kannel & McGee 1979). This latter finding, which has been confirmed in

Table 3.1 Effects of diabetes on the circulation

Component	Normal function	Disturbance in diabetes
Arteries		
Elastic	Carrying blood to periphery	Atherosclerosis Early — reduced blood flow capacity Late — ischaemia and gangrene
Muscular		Calcification increased rigidity of wall increased blood flow velocity
Microcirculation		
Arteriovenous anastomosis	Thermoregulation	Increased shunt flow Increased venous pressure
Arterioles	Regulation of peripheral resistance	Hyalinization Decreased autoregulation Increased resistance to flow
Capillaries	Exchange of nutrients	Early — increased permeability Late — basement membrane thickening ? reduced exchange obliteration of capillary beds
Components of vessel wall		
Nerves		Loss of vasoconstriction especially of arteriovenous anastomoses
Hormone receptors		Reduced responsiveness to catecholamines
Muscle		Reduced autoregulation
Endothelium		Reduced EDRF production Reduced prostacyclin production
Blood		
Viscocity		Increased plasma and whole blood viscosity
Oxygen delivery		Reduced availability of oxygen from haemoglobin
Coagulation		
Fluid phase		Decreased endogenous heparin activity Decreased antithrombin III activity Increased fibrinogen Increased factor VIII activity
Platelet		Various changes. See text for details

other studies, is of particular interest because it shows that diabetic women lose the relative immunity from vascular disease that non-diabetic women enjoy. It is important to note that the variation in susceptibility to arterial disease between different populations is only partly explained by risk factors attributable to the presence of diabetes (West et al 1983). It is likely that genetic and/or environmental factors play a major role.

The risk of coronary artery disease also applies to people who are hyperglycaemic but not frankly diabetic. Criteria for the diagnosis of diabetes

(National Diabetes Data Group 1979) include impaired glucose tolerance. In a study of English civil servants (Fuller et al 1980) subjects with blood glucose levels of $\geq$ 5.37 mmol/l had a coronary heart disease mortality at 7.5 years of the same order as that of known diabetics and twice that of people with lower blood glucose levels. However this group of patients with impaired glucose tolerance did not develop the microvascular complications. In a similar community study in Bedford UK, the mortality from all causes was increased in hyperglycaemic women and much of this increase appeared to be due to an excess of deaths from coronary heart disease (Jarrett et al 1982). However, it should be noted that there was no statistically significant increase in mortality in men. In addition, there is evidence that the prevalence of leg ischaemia may not be increased in patients with impaired glucose tolerance (Vaccaro et al 1985).

Another approach has been to study prevalence of glucose intolerance in patients with symptomatic arterial disease. Wahlberg (1966) and Epstein (1967) have demonstrated that abnormalities of glucose tolerance occur more frequently than normal in patients with either coronary or peripheral vascular disease. One problem has been to determine if the observed abnormalities in glucose tolerance resulted from an episode of, for example, myocardial infarction. However, it has been shown that hyperglycaemia occurs in patients with coronary or peripheral arterial disease who do not have infarction or gangrene.

The frequency with which disease occurs and the earlier stages of the natural history of atherosclerosis affecting the leg have seldom been studied. Marinelli et al (1979) used non-invasive techniques for assessing the presence of arterial disease in a large prospective study of diabetics. They found that one third of the patients without a history of intermittent claudication had evidence of arterial disease on testing. One fifth of the subjects with normal physical findings had abnormal results to these tests. In a subsequent report (Beach et al 1982), atherosclerosis in the lower limb of Type 2 (non-insulin-dependent) patients was 20 times more common than in age- and sex-matched controls. Furthermore, in patients with detectable disease, progression occurred in 87% over a period of 2 years and 22% of patients died during the follow-up period (Beach et al 1988).

Autopsy evidence

Shortly after the discovery of insulin, it was noted that many deaths in diabetic patients were due to arterial disease. The evidence from autopsy studies (e.g. Bell 1950), which showed that diabetics frequently died of vascular disease, has been criticized because of the difficulties in ensuring that the sample studied were representative (clearly patients undergoing autopsy are a specially selected sample) and in describing a high prevalence of one common disease in the presence of another. However the autopsy evidence from a major international study suggests that patients with diabetes have an increased risk of developing atherosclerosis (Robertson & Strong 1968).

Pathology

The fully developed atherosclerotic plaque comprises an irregular lumpy thickening of the artery wall. Qualitatively, the changes in diabetics are similar to those in non-diabetics. The process first affects the innermost layer of the wall, the tunica intima, where accumulations of lipid-filled cells occur. They appear macroscopically as 'fatty streaks' and may be found in young adults. They are associated with thickening and increased fibrosis in the tunica intima. As the process extends the tunica media becomes involved. Vascular smooth muscle cells proliferate and fibrosis increases. Large amounts of extracellular lipid and cholesterol are probably derived from the lipid-filled cells seen at the earlier stage. Progression of the lesion may result in destruction of the elastic fibres and weakening of the wall. Finally, the intima over the plaque may necrose resulting in the discharge of atheromatous material into the arterial tree as emboli. If released into the cerebral circulation this material may cause strokes or transient ischaemic attacks. Haemorrhage into a plaque may precipitate rupture. Ulceration which follows this process predisposes to platelet aggregation and thrombus formation. Small platelet aggregates may break off as emboli. Thrombosis may cause occlusion of the artery.

Aetiology

The most popular theory of atherogenesis at present cites injury to the endothelium as the initiating cause. The injury may be mechanical, e.g. hypertension; or chemical, e.g. hyperlipidaemia or hypertriglyceridaemia. There are a number of consequences which follow this injury of which the most important are adherence of monocytes, an increased permeability to lipids and platelet aggregation. For details of current ideas on the pathogenesis of atherosclerosis see Ross (1986).

There is much current interest in the observation that low-density lipoproteins, when circulating in high concentration, may start a vicious circle of endothelial injury and lipid accummulation. Smooth muscle cells and/or fibroblasts are stimulated by a number of factors which are released from platelets. One of these, platelet-derived growth factor, has been used to promote wound healing (see page 70). The effects of these substances may be enhanced by increasing the activity of cAMP as a consequence of adrenaline and AMP release from activated platelets. The early changes may be reversible but the persistence of various risk factors, e.g. hyperlipidaemia, causes many lesions to progress.

The detailed mechanisms are very complex and not fully understood. Figure 3.1 shows a simplified account of these events; it does not indicate

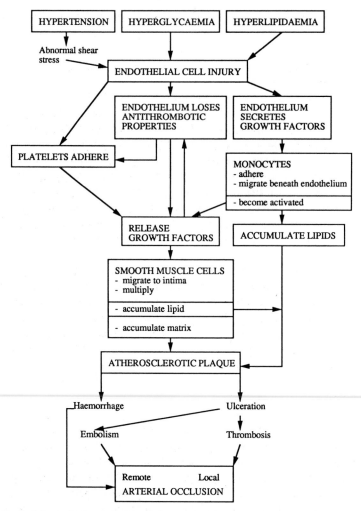

Fig. 3.1 Aetiology of atherosclerosis.

the action of smoking, genetic, environmental and hormonal factors though each of these is a major determinant of the development of atherosclerosis.

The mechanisms by which diabetes causes the accelerated development of atherosclerosis are not certain although many possibilities have been investigated and the topic has been reviewed by Ganda (1980).

Blood lipids

The biochemistry of blood lipids is complex; sophisticated analytical methods are required for many of the measurements. For this reason there have been difficulties in accumulating epidemiological data relating blood lipids to arterial disease in diabetes. The available evidence suggests that there may be different determinants of disease in the coronary and peripheral circulation in diabetic patients (West et al 1983). For example, serum lipids are significantly related to the presence of coronary artery disease but not to leg vascular disease, which is more influenced by hyperglycaemia and duration of diabetes.

Abnormalities in blood lipids can be demonstrated in about half the diabetic population. This figure varies with the age of the patient, the type of diabetes and the control of blood glucose. In addition to the increased concentrations of low density lipoproteins mentioned above, Type 2 diabetics (but not Type 1 insulin-dependent diabetics) frequently have reduced concentrations of high-density lipoproteins (HDL). HDL protects against the development of atherosclerosis (Gordon et al 1977), therefore a low concentration of HDL makes diabetics more susceptible. It should be noted that not all subgroups of diabetics have reduced HDL levels (Reckless et al 1978, Beach et al 1979). Other changes which might predispose to atherosclerosis include abnormalities in the metabolism of low- and very-low-density lipoproteins and changes in the proteins (apoproteins) responsible for the carriage of lipoproteins in the blood.

It is important to note that there is good evidence that control of diabetes improves serum lipid patterns and this is likely to have an important beneficial effect on the rate of progression of arterial disease.

Hypertension

Hypertension is a risk factor for the development of atherosclerosis in non-diabetic patients and there is epidemiological evidence that blood pressure is an important predictor of atherosclerosis in diabetics (Keen 1985).

The relationship between diabetes and hypertension has been reviewed by Drury (1983). Reports on the occurrence of hypertension in diabetics vary in their conclusions. However, it appears that there is an excess of patients with systolic hypertension in both Type 1 and Type 2 diabetes. In Type 1 patients, there is an increase in hypertension above the age of 45–50, but diastolic hypertension appears to be related to the presence of nephropathy. In Type 2 patients, there is little evidence of increased diastolic hypertension. Systolic hypertension in these subjects is largely, but not entirely, related to obesity.

There is good evidence of an association between hypertension and retinopathy, but no evidence that controlling hypertension slows the progress of the vascular disease. On the other hand, control of hypertension has been shown to slow the deterioration in glomerular filtration rate in patients with nephropathy.

The mechanisms whereby diabetics become hypertensive are not fully understood, but there is evidence that excess insulin may increase sodium reabsorption by the kidney. Other mechanisms include altered sensitivity of the blood vessels to circulating vasoconstricor substances, e.g. angiotension II and catecholamines.

Hyperglycaemia

Hyperglycaemia was shown to be an independent risk factor for the development of atherosclerosis in the Framingham and Busselton (Western Australia) community studies. There is evidence from prevalence studies that there is a range of risks between groups with normal, borderline and clearly abnormal glucose metabolism. The possible mechanisms include impairment of vessel wall metabolism or nutrition, changes in coagulation, or osmotic effects. Hyperglycaemia may also have a direct stimulatory effect on the smooth muscle cell. It should be noted that blood glucose concentration is statistically associated with a number of other factors which are related to the development of arterial disease (Keen et al 1981). These include age, blood pressure, obesity, plasma lipids and plasma insulin. It is not known if the association between atherosclerosis and hyperglycaemia is direct or via some other factor (West et al 1983).

Hyperinsulinism

There is evidence that increased circulating levels of insulin may be a cause of atherosclerosis (Stout 1981, Ledet 1981, Stolar 1988) although Jarrett (1988) considers the case 'not proven'. Hyperinsulinism may act independently of raised serum lipids or hypertension, and it can be demonstrated that atherosclerotic non-diabetic patients have elevated insulin secretion in response to oral glucose. This response may predict the development of coronary artery disease. In Type 2 diabetic subjects there is evidence that insulin levels are increased and there is evidence that in Type 1 diabetics the insulin requirements are greater than the normal daily secretion of the pancreas.

There are several possible mechanisms by which excess insulin may accelerate the development of atherosclerosis and there have been a number of experiments to show that insulin promotes the changes associated with the development of atherosclerosis. These mechanisms include increased accummulation of lipid and increased incorporation of glucose into lipids in the arterial wall, stimulation of proliferation of smooth muscle cells, increased uptake and synthesis of lipid by these cells and the inhibition of fibrinolysis. It is suggested that an important aim of therapy in Type 2 diabetics should be to minimize hyperinsulinaemia (Stolar 1988).

Blood coagulation

There have been a number of observations on blood coagulation mechanisms which point to the existence of a hypercoagulable state in diabetes.

Through increased deposition of fibrin this could accelerate the development of atherosclerotic plaques (see Jones & Peterson 1981 for review). Reported abnormalities include decreased endogenous heparin and antithrombin activity, elevation of factor VIII activity, and increased plasma fibrinogen concentrations (especially in patients with vascular disease). There have been conflicting or inconclusive reports on the concentrations of antithrombin III and the activity of the fibrinolytic system. However, there is evidence of increased turnover and reduced survival of fibrinogen which is consistent with a hypercoagulable state. The abnormalities in the activity of the platelets are discussed in the section on microangiopathy (see page 34).

Mechanical factors

There has been recent interest in physical factors that might determine the characteristic distribution of atheroma at the branch points of arteries. It can be shown that at these sites the endothelium is thicker, the cell turnover more rapid and the endothelium is abnormally permeable to protein. The walls of arteries are stiffer in diabetic patients as a consequence of accumulation of type IV collagen. The stiffness is enhanced by glycosylation of the collagen. This stiffening, in addition to hypertension and increased viscosity, will increase the shear stress in the wall at these points. The hypothesis is that the endothelium is damaged by the shear stresses and thus becomes more permeable to the lipoproteins which may be circulating in increased amounts in diabetic patients. This initiates atherogenesis.

Smoking

Cigarette smoking is strongly associated with the development of atherosclerosis. The mechanism is uncertain but it may be related to changes in the permeability of the wall to proteins. In diabetic subjects an important interaction between diabetes and cigarette smoking accounted for 65% of cardiovascular deaths in one community survey (Suarez & Barrett-Connor 1984, Masarei et al 1986).

Morphology and distribution

The macroscopic features of streaks and plaques of atheroma are indistinguishable in diabetics and non-diabetics but there is good evidence that the distribution of the disease is different. In the leg, the distribution of atherosclerosis has been studied by arteriography and examination of amputation specimens. In non-diabetics the common patterns of disease are as follows:

Occlusion of the femoral artery. This is the most common lesion and characteristically starts at the region of the hiatus in the adductor magnus muscle where the femoral artery passes close to the femur. Extension of the occlusion to involve the whole length of the superficial femoral artery is common.

Stenosis or occlusion of the aorta and/or iliac arteries. This may occur at any level from the origin of the renal arteries (from the aorta) to the inguinal ligament. Stenosis of the iliac arteries may be difficult to see on arteriograms taken in a single anteroposterior plane because the disease commonly forms a plaque along the posterior wall of the iliac artery.

Stenosis of the profunda femoris artery. This vessel, which is the major source of blood for the thigh muscles, is often affected by atheroma which causes narrowing at its origin. Such narrowing can be demonstrated in about 20% of patients with leg ischaemia. In a patient with obstruction of the femoral artery, this stenosis is sometimes treated instead of performing a bypass operation. More commonly it is corrected as part of an aorto-femoral reconstruction.

Diffuse disease. In addition to the patterns described, atherosclerosis may cause any combination of stenosis or occlusion of the arteries between the aorta and the ankle. Diabetic patients may exhibit any of these patterns of disease but the characteristic pattern is of disease which becomes more severe in the more distal parts of the limb. The angiographic pattern of disease seen in diabetic patients has the following features (Figs. 3.2–3.5):

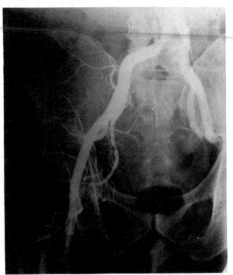

Fig. 3.2

Figs. 3.2–3.5 Arteriogram showing the typical pattern of atherosclerosis associated with diabetes. The iliac arteries (3.2) and the upper part of the femoral artery (3.3) are patent. In the popliteal artery (3.4) there is a stenosing plaque of atheroma at the level of the intercondylar notch of the femur. The arteries of the calf (3.5) are very severely diseased. There is no possibility of improving the circulation by performing arterial surgery in such a limb.

1. The aorta and iliac arteries are patent and show only minor areas of irregularity in the wall.

2. The common and superficial arteries are patent. There may be areas of narrowing in the superficial femoral artery. These are more severe distally in the thigh.

3. The profunda femoris artery may be irregularly narrowed in its distal part.

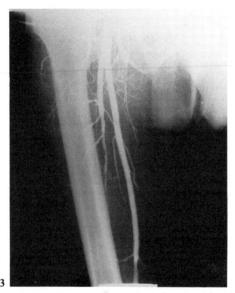

Fig. 3.3

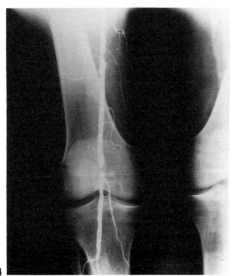

Fig. 3.4

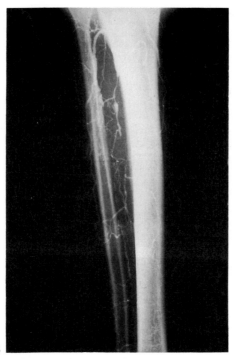

Fig. 3.5

4. The proximal part of the popliteal artery is often patent but the distal part is frequently occluded.

5. The tibial arteries are severely diseased. There may be no identifiable named calf arteries (Fig. 3.5) or only one of the three major calf arteries (usually the peroneal artery) may be seen.

6. The major pedal vessels are not severely affected.

From the point of view of treatment, the most serious feature of this pattern is the occlusion of the distal popliteal artery and its distal branches (Strandness et al 1964). This makes arterial reconstructive surgery more difficult because the distal end of an arterial bypass is placed beyond the area of occlusion. This means that in many diabetic patients the anastomosis must be performed to tibial vessels and this may be a difficult technical exercise.

Disease in the arteries of the foot has seldom been studied. There are several possible reasons for this including the difficulty of performing arteriography on the foot arteries and the inability to treat disease of these vessels. However, if the tendency for arterial occlusion to affect the distal vessels is extended from the calf to the foot, this might have important implications for the healing in local areas of injury and might predispose to the spread of necrosis.

Figs. 3.6–3.7 Disease in small arteries.

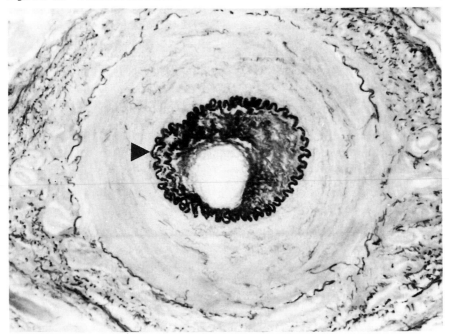

Fig. 3.6 The internal elastic lamina (arrow) encloses an eccentrically-thickened tunica intima.

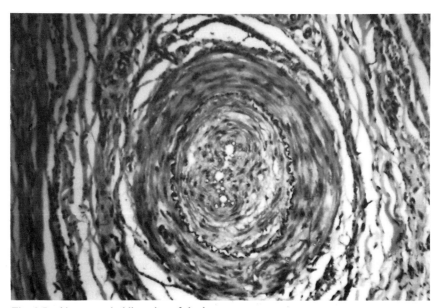

Fig. 3.7 Almost total obliteration of the lumen.

Foot arteriography has shown that there may be hypervascularity and appearances suggesting microaneurysm formation. In a study by Ferrier (1967) the histological appearances were of a uniform, although often asymmetrical, thickening of the tunica intima (Figs 3.6–3.7). This contrasted with the lumpy appearance of atheromatous plaques in larger arteries. The diseased intima comprised a loose collagen network with pale ground substance and few nuclei. It did not stain with periodic acid-Schiff stain and did not contain elastic fibres. These changes were qualitatively similar in both diabetics and non-diabetics. The metatarsal arteries were, however, more often obstructed in diabetics. The nature of this disease is unknown but it is important because it demonstrates that arterial disease is contiguous from the aorta to the capillaries.

CALCIFICATION OF ARTERIES

Calcification of the tunica media of muscular arteries is a common feature of longstanding diabetes, which is the commonest cause of these changes. Arterial calcification may result from deposition of calcium salts either in atheromatous plaques of the tunica intima, e.g. in the wall of an aortic aneurysm, or in the tunica media. Calcification in the tunica intima, which is common in atherosclerosis, has an irregular lumpy appearance on radiographs. In contrast, calcification of the tunica media may be distinguishable because of its relatively regular, fine, speckled appearance (Figs. 3.8–3.9). In addition medial calcification commonly affects the vessels of the foot which are seldom affected by atherosclerosis.

Several studies have demonstrated that medial calcification is more common in diabetics. Its frequency has been related to age, male sex and duration of diabetes in those aged less than 50 years. Neubauer (1971) made the observation that calcification of the vessels of non-diabetics was related to higher levels of blood glucose following a glucose load. This suggests that hyperglycaemia has a direct role in the development of this condition and in this regard it is similar to atherosclerosis.

The aetiology of these changes is uncertain. Evidence has been produced to suggest that neuropathy is a cause. It has been found that calcification is more closely related to neuropathy than to microangiopathy (Edmonds et al 1982, Corbin et al 1987). In patients with neuropathic joints, which are an important manifestation of neuropathy, calcification is also more common. Histologically the calcification starts in senescent smooth muscle and sympathectomy may cause foci of degeneration of smooth muscle. The alternative hypothesis is that the muscle damage is part of widespread changes in connective tissue occurring in diabetics.

Arterial calcification has been used as a prognostic indicator in diabetics (Everhart et al 1988). They found that the incidence of nephropathy, retinopathy and coronary artery disease were all increased. Most striking was a fivefold increase in the chances of amputation. However, the effects of calcified vessels on the blood supply to the foot remains uncertain. It has been demonstrated that arterial calcification is associated with a reduction in the peak blood flow which is an index of the capacity of the circulation to increase. This alone would probably have only a minor effect on the blood supply to the foot. It has also been demonstrated that advanced vascular calcification is associated with narrowing or occlusion arising in the tunica intima. On the other hand, the tunica intima may be relatively unaffected despite major deposits of calcium in the tunica media (see Fig. 3.10).

One important practical point is that calcification of the tunica media makes the wall of the artery difficult to compress so that measurement of the blood pressure by external compression of an artery will be less accurate. This problem is discussed later (see page 140). This phenomenon is well recognized but there is no reliable information about the frequency with which it occurs.

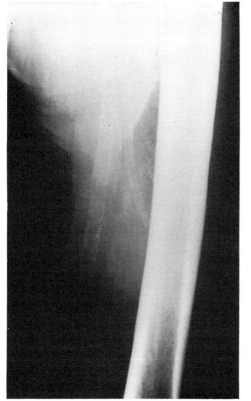 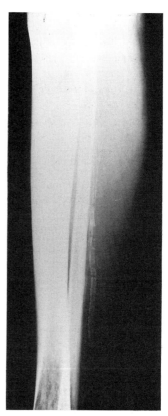

Fig. 3.8   **Fig. 3.9**

Figs. 3.8–3.9   Radiograph of thigh (3.8) and calf (3.9) showing very extensive calcification of large arteries. In the thigh the superficial and deep femoral arteries can be clearly identified. The fine regular pattern suggests that the calcification is in the tunica media.

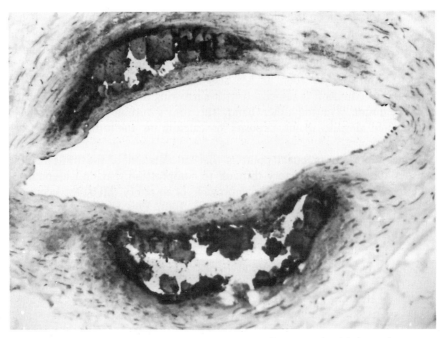

Fig. 3.10 Arterial calcification Section through a muscular artery showing large plaques of calcification. The tunica intima is normal.

MICROANGIOPATHY

Two of the major causes of morbidity in diabetics, namely retinopathy and nephropathy, have been known for many years to be due to microvascular disease. A hypothesis that disease of the microscopic blood vessels might be the cause of the major complications was suggested by Dry & Hines (1941) who noted the clinical association between retinopathy, neuropathy and nephropathy and suggested that the common factor was disease of the small blood vessels. This reinforced the assumption that small vessel disease was also important in the development of foot lesions.

Two reports in 1959 mark the beginning of modern research into the morphology and function of small vessels in diabetes. Goldenberg et al (1959) described changes in the small vessels of amputated limbs which they believed to be characteristic of diabetes. Fagerberg (1959) studied the small vessels in biopsy specimens from the sural nerve and considered that the changes he saw were the cause of the neuropathy.

The changes, which are typical if not pathognomonic of diabetes, can be divided into two histological groups. The importance of these findings has been re-evaluated in recent years and it is now believed that the proliferative changes described by Goldenberg et al are less important and less specific than was formerly thought.

1. Thickening of capillary basement membranes

These changes are the hallmark of diabetic microangiopathy. When seen with the light microscope (Fig. 3.11) the appearance is of focal thickening of the vessel wall. The staining reactions of these areas indicate the presence of glycoprotein. These changes have a patchy distribution and are believed to have a common origin with renal and retinal vascular disease. On electron microscopy, laminar thickening of the capillary basement membrane is seen and this is accompanied by changes in the nuclei of the perivascular cells.

In the limbs, these changes have been seen in the skin, subcutaneous tissue, muscle and nerves. Much research has been carried out on their identification because they have been considered to be an important marker of complications of diabetes. The time at which they develop has aroused much controversy. This began with the report that basement membrane thickening in skeletal muscle capillaries was present in patients who were genetically likely to develop diabetes and in patients with latent diabetes. It was suggested that these changes might be genetically determined. However, subsequent workers have been unable to confirm these findings and much of the subsequent disagreement has hinged on the precise techniques used in preparing and examining the specimens. A majority view would now be that capillary basement membrane thickening follows, rather than precedes, the development of the metabolic derangement of diabetes (see Williamson & Kilo 1979 for summary of arguments). Although these changes are characteristic of diabetes they are not exclusive to it because

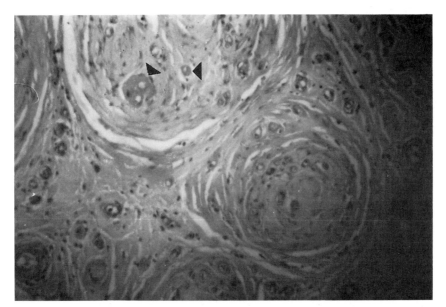

Fig. 3.11 Microangiopathy. PAS stain (X330). Section of a digital nerve from a toe. There are several capillaries showing marked thickening of the basement membrane.

identical changes have been seen in a small proportion of specimens from non-diabetics.

2. *Proliferative changes in arterioles and arteries*

These findings include (1) enlargement and proliferation of endothelial cells which might result in occlusion of vessels, (2) concentric rings of periodic acid-Schiff-positive staining material between which are enlarged endothelial cells, (3) single and intact internal elastic lamina and (4) normal tunica media. In the initial report of Goldenberg et al (1959) these changes were described in vessels up to the size of the digital arteries and, like the capillary basement membrane thickening, they could be seen in some specimens from non-diabetics, They have been identfied in many tissues from the limbs, including skin, muscle, nerve and vasa vasorum. There is some doubt if these changes represent a specific form of vascular disease or if they are merely reactive, for example, obliterative changes in vessels whose capillary beds have been reduced in size.

Functions of the microcirculation

The primary functions of the microcirculation are to transport nutrients to the peripheral tissues and remove waste products, and to assist in thermoregulation. The application of modern methods of study of the circulation has provided a greatly increased understanding of the effects of diabetes on the peripheral circulation. This has led to hypotheses to explain the development of the histological changes. The system is very complex involving structural elements of the vessel wall, the blood and external factors, such as the nervous system and circulating hormones.

The blood flow to an organ or tissue is affected by the perfusion pressure and the vascular resistance (Table 3.2A). The perfusion pressure is determined by the arteriovenous pressure difference, and the vascular resistance by the viscosity of the blood and the radius of the vessels. The vessel radius is most important because the blood flow depends on a power function of the radius (in an ideal fluid the fourth power is applicable). Thus very small changes in radius will have substantial effects on flow. Factors affecting the vessel radius are shown in Table 3.2B. They include circulating hormones, vasoconstrictor neurones and local mechanisms intrinsic to the vascular smooth muscle. The factors affecting local perfusion pressure and viscosity are shown in Table 3.2C and 3.2D respectively. All these factors affect blood flow in the capillaries. Exchange across the capillaries is dependent on the functions described previously plus factors which are intrinsic to the capillary and blood (Table 3.2E).

The functions of the microcirculation may be affected by:
1. Haemodynamic changes affecting the blood flow and pressure in the peripheral circulation.

2. Changes in the vessel wall which may cause impairment of flow, alterations in the transfer of substances across the wall, or changes to the responsiveness of the wall to various stimuli.

3. Changes in the blood which may affect the availability of oxygen in the tissues, the blood flow or the blood coagulation.

Table 3.2 Factors affecting function of the microcirculation

A. Blood flow $= \dfrac{\Delta P}{R}$

  $R = \dfrac{\text{viscosity} \times \text{length}}{(\text{radius})^n}$

B. Factors affecting vessel radius
  (i) Physiological:
    Extrinsic:
      nerves
      circulating hormones
    Intrinsic:
      local nervous mechanisms
      local vasoactive agents
      myogenic responses

  (ii) Pathological:
    Occlusion of vessels:
      platelet microthrombi
      ? proliferative changes in endothelium
    Thickening of vessel wall
    Rigidity of vessel walls:
      less response to physiological stimuli

C. Factors affecting pressure
  Arteriolar pressure:
    local arterial pressure reduced in atherosclerosis
  Arteriolar function and disease:
    (see factors affecting vessel radius)
  Venular pressure:
    increased with AV shunting

D. Factors affecting viscosity
  Red cells:
    deformability
  Plasma:
    fibrinogen concentration

E. Factors affecting exchange across capillaries
  Capillary blood flow:
    See sections B,C,D
  Capillary surface area
  Capillary filtration pressure
    (difference between intravascular and tissue pressure)
  Capillary wall thickness and permeability:
    basement membrane thickening
    chemical change
  Erythrocyte function
    Glycosylated haemoglobin
    2,3-DPG

Aetiology of microangiopathy

Haemodynamic changes

An increase in the blood flow is characteristically found early in diabetes in the kidney, retina and limb. It has been postulated that this is a cause of capillary hypertension and microvascular damage. The cause of the increased flow is uncertain but, in the limbs, several factors are known which may contribute:

1. An increase in the metabolic rate which occurs in imperfectly controlled diabetes. This requires that more heat be lost from the body and this is effected by one of the normal mechanisms, namely, an increase in blood flow to the skin.

2. There may be a chronic increase in the plasma and extracellular fluid volume.

3. There may be alterations in the action of circulating vasoactive substances:
   a. Decreased plasma renin activity
   b. Decreased sensitivity of blood vessels to angiotension II
   c. Decreased responsiveness to noradrenaline.

4. Increased production of vasodilator substances prostacylin and prostaglandin E (see below).

5. Hyperglycaemia and increased levels of glucagon and growth hormone may cause vasodilatation.

6. Tissue hypoxia, however induced, will cause local vasodilatation. This may be the step which causes accentuation in the severity of the disease (Editorial 1977, Ditzel 1980).

7. Denervation as a result of autonomic neuropathy will cause vasodilatation.

It is probable that increased blood flow through arteriovenous (AV) shunts is an important mechanism for hyperperfusion in the limbs. AV shunts are present in the digits and palmar surfaces of hands and feet. They are 20–70 micron in diameter and, when open, provide a low-resistance pathway between small arteries and veins. Their diameter is controlled by the sympathetic nervous system. If the vasoconstrictor nerves fail to function there will be a loss of autonomic control of the vascular sphincter mechanisms which regulate flow through these shunts. An increase in AV shunt blood flow will have important effects on capillary function. It will result in:

1. Reduced capillary blood flow due to:
   a. Reduced pressure at the arteriolar end of the capillary ('stealing' of blood by the shunts) and/or
   b. Increased pressure in the post-capillary venules which would

reduce the perfusion pressure (see Table 3.2C). This change would
also result in:
2. Increased in filtration pressure across the capillary wall.

There is some evidence from direct measurement that capillary blood flow
is reduced in poorly controlled diabetics (Tooke 1986), but Flynn et al
(1988) demonstrated that capillary flow was increased in diabetic neuropathic patients. There are several lines of evidence which indicate that increased shunting occurs in the lower limb in diabetics. These include, a
raised PO_2 in venous blood (Boulton et al 1982), rapid passage of microspheres from arterial to venous blood (Partsh 1977), and abnormal
sonagram tracings from foot vessels, indicating the presence of a high
diastolic blood flow or reduced peripheral resistance (Edmonds et al 1982,
Corbin et al 1988). This shunting results in a raised foot blood flow (Faris
1979) so that the foot is warm and the veins distended (Ward et al 1983).
This AV shunting has been suggested as the cause of most of the complications seen in the neuropathic foot. In experimental animals AV shunting
can cause ulcers (Neilubowicz et al 1975).

Increased blood flow may cause increased pressure in capillaries. This
may be the common pathway which leads to structural changes in the capillaries. Direct measurement of capillary blood pressure by micropuncture
of nailfold capillaries in diabetic patients has shown a normal pressure when
supine but an increase in pressure in the dependent foot (Tooke 1980,
Rayman et al 1986). This could be produced either by arteriovenous shunting as described above or by loss of the local vasoconstrictor reflex (which
causes arteriolar constriction in response to venous distension as occurs with
standing). This response is mediated through sympathetic nerve fibres which
degenerate early in the course of diabetic neuropathy. The relationship to
postural change may explain why the capillary basement membrane thickening is more pronounced in more distal parts of the limb (Vracko 1970).
Microscopy of small vessels in conjunctiva and nailfold shows that a characteristic series of changes are present. These include dilatation, elongation
and tortuosity of capillaries and venules. The most severe changes have been
associated with rapidly progressive retinopathy (Ditzel 1980).

Reduced perfusion may be demonstrated in two sets of circumstances.
Later in the disease it may be seen as a reduction in maximum blood flow.
This is important because it indicates that the tissues may not be able to
respond adequately to trauma or infection and thus failure of wound healing
may occur. There are two mechanisms for this reduction in flow. First, it
is the characteristic finding in patients with early obstruction to large
arteries, e.g. by atherosclerosis. Second, studies of local blood flow have
indicated that the flow may be reduced despite the presence of a normal
local perfusion pressure (Faris & Lassen 1982, Duncan & Faris 1986).
These haemodynamic findings have been correlated with histological

evidence of microvascular disease (Kastrup et al 1987). A reduction in retinal blood flow is also seen in patients with severe retinopathy and is a characteristic feature in patients with clinical nephropathy. These changes probably result from obstruction to the blood flow because of narrowing of the lumen by disease of the vessel wall.

In patients with diabetes of recent onset a number of haemodynamic abnormalities can be demonstrated. These suggest that there is a reduction in maximal blood flow capacity. The observations have included a reduced transcutaneous oxygen tension (Ewald et al 1981), reduced blood flow velocity in nailfold capillaries following ischaemia (Fagrell et al 1984), reduced vasodilatation in skin following heating or needle trauma (see Tooke 1986 for details) and a reduction in peak muscle blood flow following exercise (Faris et al 1982a). Other haemodynamic abnormalities which can be demonstrated include a loss of autoregulation. This is the local response of the circulation which tends to keep blood flow constant in the face of changes in perfusion pressure. Loss of this function can be demonstrated in several vascular beds including brain, kidney and skin (Faris et al 1983) (see Fig. 3.12). The mechanisms for these changes are not certain but they are consistent with changes in smooth muscle function and/or rigidity of vessel walls.

Changes in the wall

Basement membrane.   Capillary basement membrane thickening may develop as a consequence of change in the chemical environment which results in abnormal glycosylation of collagen (see Ch. 6) and/or it may represent the response of the capillary wall to injury or increased pressure as discussed above. The basic constituent of the capillary basement membrane is type IV collagen; proteoglycans, laminin and fibronectin are also present. These are normal components of connective tissue. Collagen provides the basic structure. The proteoglycans are negatively charged and may resist the filtration of similarly charged molecules in blood, e.g. albumin. Thickening of the basement membrane may be a proliferative response to injury to the capillary. There is evidence of increased synthesis and reduced degradation of basement membrane. The latter may be due to glycosylation of basement membrane collagen making it more resistant to enzymic digestion. Paradoxically, basement membrane thickening may result in an increase in the permeability characteristics due either to changes in the arrangement of the molecules or to a reduction in the number of negatively charged molecules. In addition the vessels will be more rigid and less able to respond to haemodynamic changes.

Endothelial cells.   The concept of the endothelial cells has changed dramatically in recent years. Formerly regarded as the passive lining of the blood vessels, the endothelial cell is now known to be highly active and important in regulating vascular tone, permeability and blood coagulation.

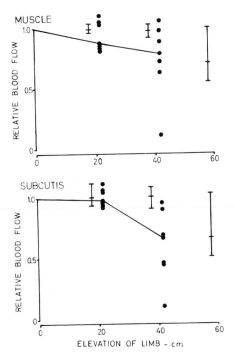

Fig. 3.12 Relative blood flow against height of elevation of the limb for muscle (left) and subcutaneous tissue (right). The vertical bars represent the range and median bars for eight normal subjects. The lines join the median values for the diabetic subjects. There is a greater fall in blood flow at 40 cm elevation in diabetics. This indicates impaired autoregulation.

Several changes in endothelial cell function have been described in diabetic subjects:

1. Decrease in prostacyclin (PgI_2) production. This substance is a potent vasodilator and acts to inhibit platelet aggregation. There is general agreement that PgI_2 production from the endothelium in arteries and veins is reduced in diabetes.

2. Endothelium dependent relaxing factor (EDRF). This substance has an important effect in regulating the contraction of vascular smooth muscle. Its activity is probably decreased in diabetes and this might cause an alteration of the responses of the vessel wall to various stimuli, e.g. circulating catecholamines. Production of EDRF has been shown to be decreased in penile smooth muscle from diabetics. This may be a factor contributing to impotence in these patients (de Tejada et al 1989).

3. Increased release of von Willebrand factor (VWF). Increased circulating levels of VWF are found in diabetics and this probably reflects endothelial damage. The levels are highest in non-insulin-dependent diabetes mellitus and in non-diabetics with

atherosclerosis. It is not clear whether this substance has any direct action in increasing blood coagulation in these patients although it may enhance platelet adhesion to subendothelial tissues.

4. Fibrinolysis. The fibrinolytic system opposes and is in balance with the blood coagulation system. One of the important components of fibrinolysis is plasminogen activator which converts plasminogen to plasmin and is produced by the endothelium. The level of plasminogen activator in the vessel wall is low in diabetics and may be depressed further by circulating inhibitors. This might tend to promote thrombosis but its exact effect is uncertain.

One important group of consequences of these changes is an increase in permeability of the capillary wall. This can be demonstrated for water, large molecules, e.g. albumin, and smaller molecules, e.g. fluorescein and has led to one of the major hypotheses for the development of microangiopathy. This is that the increased permeability to substance like albumin and IgG results in the deposition of these substances in the blood vessel wall (Parving 1976). This is the concept of hyaline changes or plasmatic vasculosis. It is supported by the demonstration that many different plasma proteins are present in the vessel wall, including albumin, IgG, IgM and fibrin (Cohn et al 1978).

The escape of albumin into the urine is an important marker of nephropathy and is aggravated by hypertension. Reduction in blood pressure can reduce the amount of proteinuria (Parving et al 1985). It has been demonstrated that albumin is deposited in the basement membrane of blood vessels in the skin (Chavers et al 1981), and albumin or IgG in muscle capillaries. The permeability to water and hydrophilic ions is also increased. This suggests that basement membrane thickening does not limit the rate of transport of these substances. Recent studies in which skin capillaries were examined directly after intravenous injection of fluoroscein have demonstrated an increased permeability of diabetic capillaries to this substance (Bollinger et al 1982). This result is best explained by the enhanced diffusion across less effective barriers.

The possible effect of changes in the basement membrane has been discussed earlier. The cause of these changes in permeability remains unclear. However, increased permeability could result from altered surface charge density of endothelial cells, damaged intercellular junctions or increased transcellular transport (Williamson & Kilo 1983).

Changes in the blood

There are three groups of changes in the blood which might impede flow in the microcirculation. These are changes in viscosity, which cause increased resistance to blood flow, and an increased coagulability which results from an imbalance between the procoagulant and anticoagulant activities of platelets and vascular endothelium.

Change in viscosity. The viscosity of blood can be described in terms of either plasma viscosity or whole blood viscosity. Both are increased in diabetics, resulting in an increased resistance to blood flow and therefore a reduction in volume flow. This effect could be potentiated in an area of decreased pressure distal to an arterial obstruction. In recent years it has been realized that red blood cells change shape as they pass through capillaries which are narrower in diameter than the red blood cells. This property is called deformability of red cells. In diabetes the cells are more rigid and therefore less able to traverse small capillaries. This abnormality is lessened by the administration of insulin (Vague & Juhan 1983).

Changes in oxygen delivery to tissues. Relative hypoxia may result from an increased metabolic rate in the tissues (p. 28) or from a reduction in oxygen delivery. The latter may be due to changes in the affinity of the haemoglobin molecule for oxygen. The oxygen dissociation curve (Fig. 3.13) may be shifted to the left in diabetic patients. This shift means that for a given oxygen tension the percent saturation is higher, i.e. more oxygen remains bound to the haemoglobin molecule therefore less is available to the tissues. Such a shift can be demonstrated acutely following the administration of insulin and the treatment of ketoacidosis and may result in a significant reduction in the amount of oxygen available to the tissues at those times.

There are several factors which might cause this shift. One of the important regulators of oxygen release by the haemoglobin molecule is 2,3-diphosphoglycerate (2,3-DPG). This byproduct of glucose metabolism

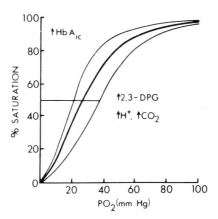

Fig. 3.13 Effect of increased concentrations of HbA Ic,2,3-DPG, H^+ and CO_2 on the oxygen dissociation curve.

reduces the affinity of haemoglobin for oxygen. The concentration in the red cells of 2,3-DPG falls during the treatment of ketosis and this may worsen the local hypoxia. This probably occurs because insulin administration decreases the concentration of plasma inorganic phosphate and this inhibits 2,3-DPG formation. In addition there may be increased amounts of haemoglobin AIc (HbA_{IC}) which has a greater affinity for oxygen and therefore also shifts the haemoglobin dissociation curve to the left. HbA_{IC} is believed to be formed by the non-enzymic addition of glucose to the end of the beta chain of the haemoglobin molecule (see p. 92 for more details). However it has been pointed out (Koenig & Cerami 1980) that mutant haemoglobin with a much greater affinity for oxygen is not associated with clinical vascular disease.

Changes in blood clotting.   A number of changes indicate that blood is more coagulable in diabetics. Changes in the fluid phase of blood coagulation have been discussed on page 16. Platelets are an essential component of the haemostatic response, the initial stages of which take place in contact with damaged endothelium or areas from which the endothelium has been lost. Thus the endothelial factors described above will have an influence on the function of platelets. However, there are a number of changes in platelet function demonstrable in diabetics before the development of clinical evidence of microangiopathy (Colwell et al 1983).

1. Platelet aggregation.   In diabetic subjects most studies have demonstrated an increase in platelet aggregation when exposed to ADP or collagen. These changes are more prominent in patients with established microvascular disease.

2. Increased thromboxane production.   These substances are the antagonists of the prostacyclin produced by the endothelium. In general the function of thromboxanes is to cause vasoconstriction and platelet aggregation. There is good evidence from experimental diabetes and patients before and after the development of microangiopathy that the production of these substances by diabetic platelets is increased.

3. Release of beta-thromboglobulin.   This protein is released into the plasma from platelets which have been activated. In most studies elevated levels have been found in patients before the development of microangiopathy. This indicates that abnormal degrees of platelet activation and release are occurring. The level is reduced after the administration of insulin.

4. Platelet survival.   A reduction in platelet survival time indicates that platelets are being activated and destroyed abnormally rapidly. It is found in diabetics before and after the development of vascular disease.

5. Platelet microthrombi.   Pathological support for the role of platelets in the development of microangiopathy has come from the demonstration that platelet microthrombi can be found in the retinal vessels of diabetic rats.

If platelets are important in causing clinical microangiopathy, it should be possible to slow the development of disease by inhibiting platelet function, e.g. with aspirin. The outcome of trials to test this hypothesis is awaited with interest. The significance of these changes in coagulability is uncertain. In the early stages of increased blood flow they are obviously not impairing the microcirculation, but in later stages, when the microvessels become narrow and rigid, the increased viscosity and coagulability might act to further reduce flow in the microcirculation and thus worsen the tissue hypoxia.

CLINICAL EFFECTS

Atherosclerosis

From the discussion of the occurrence of atherosclerosis in the diabetic leg it can be deduced that diabetics are liable to the same consequences of impairment of the blood supply to the leg as non-diabetics. Thus diabetics may develop intermittent claudication, manifesting the same signs and requiring the same treatment as non-diabetics. If the occlusion is more severe, rest pain or gangrene may occur and the clinical features and principles of treatment are identical in both diabetics and non-diabetics (see p. 176). However, the treatment may be more difficult in patients with diabetes because of the presence of atherosclerosis in the calf vessels (see p. 18).

Atherosclerotic occlusion is the major aetiological factor in about half the patients who present with foot ulcers or gangrene in Western communities with their large populations of Type 2, non-insulin-dependent diabetics. In clinics seeing many young patients or in developing countries, atherosclerosis is less common as a cause of foot lesions. The tests for the presence of atherosclerosis are discussed in Chapter 9 and include the measurement of skin perfusion pressure, ankle or toe blood pressure and angiography. Because of the frequent presence of arterial calcification in these patients, the skin perfusion pressure or toe blood pressure is preferred for assessment.

Small vessel disease

The question of whether the small vessel changes are important in causing foot lesions is one of the unresolved problems in diabetes. This question may be considered in two parts.

Digital and metatarsal arteries

Disease of these vessels is not usually considered an important factor but there are several lines of evidence that suggest an association between disease at this level and the development of foot lesions. If segmental blood pressures are measured, it is found that diabetics have a greater fall in pressure between ankle and toe than non-diabetics. This observation has been extended with the report (Faris 1975) that the highest gradients occur in those diabetics who develop foot ulcers and gangrene and this observation is independent of the presence of atherosclerosis in the leg. The pathological changes, which probably explain these observations, have been recorded by Ferrier (1967) and described previously.

Arteriolar and capillary disease

This continues to be a topic of lively debate. A major difficulty has been the inability to diagnose microvascular disease in the living limb without biopsy which is contraindicated in many of these patients. Several studies have tried to assess the importance of disease identified histologically in the development of foot lesions. Moore & Frew (1965) found a strong association between the presence of foot lesions and the finding of proliferative changes in skin vessels. Conversely, Stary (1966) believed, from his study of amputation specimens, that the changes in the larger and medium-sized arteries were sufficient to cause the skin necrosis seen. Similarly, Banson & Lacy (1964) and Conrad (1967) found that lesions of small vessels were no more serious in diabetics with gangrene than in non-diabetics. Du Plessis (1970) found capillary changes in 50% of his patients with lesions, although he did not provide any information about their frequency in control subjects. In my own series, microangiopathy could be found in about half the patients with foot ulcers. It is difficult to see how this patchy change in the smallest blood vessels could be responsible for large areas of necrosis. Nielsen (1973) found no cases with proliferative changes, and capillary changes in only four out of 15 diabetics with foot ulcers. He concluded that the microangiopathy did not cause the lesions. The evidence from these studies supports the conclusion that changes in capillaries and arterioles are probably not responsible for the development of ulcers and gangrene in diabetics.

Recent studies have examined several aspects of the function of the microcirculation in the leg in diabetics. In summary, these have demonstrated reduced vasodilator capacity in resistance vessels (Faris et al 1982), reduced capacity for autoregulation (Faris et al 1983, Kastrup et al 1985) and reduced distensibility of the microcirculation in muscle (Faris et al 1982, Fig. 3.14) and skin (Kastrup et al 1987). While these changes alone might not be sufficient to cause necrosis, they might provide increased resistance to flow, and, in series with resistance due to proximal arterial obstruction, cause reduced flow which would predispose to ulceration and gangrene or retard healing (Kastrup et al 1984).

In clinical practice patients are seen in whom the large artery supply is normal or near normal, perhaps after a bypass graft, but in whom healing of foot lesions is very slow or fails to occur despite careful local treatment. In these cases it is difficult to escape the conclusion that there is inadequacy of the distal circulation in the foot. Recently we reported the results of a radioisotope clearance test in diagnosing microvascular disease in the skin. The method is discussed later (see p. 142) and we have produced several

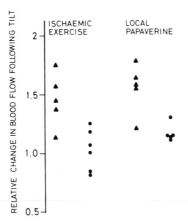

Fig. 3.14 Relative blood flow after tilt Left panel after ischaemic exercise, right panel after local papaverine. Normal subjects (▲), diabetics (●). The reduced response in the diabetic subjects indicates reduced distensibility. From Faris et al (1982).

lines of evidence to suggest that the vascular resistance in the skin measured using this method indicates the presence of microvascular disease (see p. 50 for details). We believe that microvascular disease is an important factor in the foot lesions of 20–30% of the patients we treat and an independent factor responsible for failure of healing (Faris et al 1988).

The view which minimizes the importance of microvascular disease has been reported by LoGerfo & Coffman (1984). I agree with their view that patients should be assessed as if microvascular disease was not present, i.e. the severity of atherosclerosis should be assessed as outlined on page 134, and decisions made on the basis of that information. However, even when this has been done carefully and technically successful arterial surgery performed, when indicated, there will still be some patients in whom healing does not occur. Our evidence indicates that the presence of microangiopathy explains many of the bad results obtained.

REFERENCES

Banson B B, Lacy P E 1964 Diabetic microangiopathy in human toes. American Journal of Pathology 45: 41–58
Beach K W, Bedford G R, Bergelin R O, Martin D C, Vandenberghe N, Zaccardi M, Strandness D E 1988 Progression of lower extremity arterial occlusive disease in type II diabetes mellitus. Diabetes Care 11: 464–472
Beach K W, Brunzell J D, Conquest L L, Strandness D E 1979 The insulin-dependent and non-insulin-dependent diabetes. Diabetes 28: 836–840
Beach K W, Brunzell J D, Strandness D E 1982 Prevalence of severe arteriosclerosis obliterans in patients with diabetes mellitus. Arteriosclerosis 2: 275–280
Bell E T 1950 A postmortem study of 1214 diabetic subjects with special reference to the vascular lesions. Proceedings of the American Diabetes Association 10: 62–82
Bollinger A, Frey J, Jager K, Furrer J, Seglias J, Siegenthaler W 1982 Patterns of diffusion through skin capillaries in patients with long-term diabetes. New England Journal of Medicine 307: 1305–1310

Boulton J M, Scarpello J H B, Ward J D 1982 Venous oxygenation in the diabetic neuropathic foot: evidence for arteriovenous shunting? Diabetologia 22: 6–8

Chavers B, Etzwiler D, Michael A F 1981 Albumin deposition in dermal capillary basement membrane in insulin-dependent diabetes mellitus: a preliminary report. Diabetes 30: 275–278

Cohn R A, Mauer S M, Barbosa J, Michael A F 1978 Immunofluorescence studies of skeletal muscle extracellular membranes in diabetes mellitus. Laboratory Investigation 39: 13–16

Colwell J A, Winocour P D, Halushka P V 1983 Do platelets have anything to do with diabetic microvascular disease? Diabetes 32 (suppl 2 pt 2): 14–19

Conrad M C 1967 Large and small artery occlusion in diabetics and non-diabetics with severe vascular disease. Circulation 36: 83–91

Corbin D O C, Young R J, Morrison D C, Hoskins P, McDicken W N, Housley E, Clarke B F 1987 Blood flow in the foot, polyneuropathy and foot ulceration in diabetes mellitus. Diabetologia 30: 468–473.

de Tejada I S, Goldstein I, Azadozi K, Krane R J, Cohen R A 1989. Impaired neurogenic and endothelium-mediated relaxation of penile smooth muscle from diabetic men with impotence. New England Journal of Medicine 320: 1025–1030.

Ditzel J 1980 Affinity hypoxia as a pathogenic factor of microangiopathy with particular reference to diabetic retinopathy. Acta Endocrinologia 94 (suppl): 39–55

Drury P L 1983 Diabetes and arterial hypertension. Diabetologia 24: 1–9

Dry T J, Hines E A 1941 The role of diabetes in the development of degenerative vascular disease with special reference to the evidence of retinitis and peripheral neuritis. Annals of Internal Medicine 14: 1893–1902

Duncan H J, Faris I 1986 Evaluation of an isotope washout technique to measure skin vascular resistance and skin perfusion pressure: influence of age, site and arterial surgery. Clinical Science 70: 249–255

Du Plessis D J 1970 Lesions on the feet in patients with diabetes mellitus. South African Journal of Surgery 8: 29–46

Editorial. Pathogenesis of Diabetic Microangiopathy. British Medical Journal 1977 1: 1555–1556

Edmonds M E, Morrison N, Laws J W, Watkins P J 1982 Medial arterial calcification and diabetic neuropathy. British Medical Journal 284: 928–930

Epstein F H 1967 Hyperglycaemia: a risk factor in coronary heart disease. Circulation 36: 609–619

Everhart J E, Pettitt D J, Knowler W C, Rose F A, Bennett P H 1988 Medial arterial calcification and its association with mortality and complications of diabetes. Diabetologia 31: 16–23

Ewald U, Tuvemo T, Rooth G 1981 Early reduction of vascular reactivity in diabetic children detected by transcutaneous oxygen electrode. Lancet 1: 1287–1288

Fagerberg S E 1959 Diabetic neuropathy. Acta Medica Scandanavica supp 345: 1–80

Fagrell B, Hermansson I-L, Karlander S-G, Ostergren J 1984 Vital capillary microscopy for assessment of skin viability and microangiopathy in patients with diabetes mellitus. Acta Medica Scandanavica 687: 25–28

Faris I 1975 Small and large vessel disease in the development of foot lesions in diabetics. Diabetologia 11: 249–253

Faris I 1979 The diabetic foot. MD Thesis Monash University, Melbourne, Australia

Faris I, Agerskov K, Henriksen O, Lassen N A, Parving H-H 1982 Decreased distensibility of a passive vascular bed in diabetes mellitus: an indicator of diabetic microangiopathy? Diabetologia 23: 411–414

Faris I, Duncan H, Young C 1988 Factors affecting outcome of diabetic patients with foot ulcers or gangrene. Journal of Cardiovascular Surgery 29: 736–740

Faris I, Lassen N A 1982 Increased vascular resistance in vasodilated skin: an indicator of diabetic microangiography? Cardiovascular Research 16: 607–609

Faris I, Nielsen H V, Henriksen O, Parving H-H, Lassen N A 1983 Impaired autoregulation of blood flow in skeletal muscle and subcutaneous tissue in long-term type 1 (insulin-dependent) diabetic patients with microangiopathy. Diabetologia 25: 486–488

Ferrier T M 1967 Comparative study of arterial disease in amputated lower limbs from diabetics and non-diabetics. Medical Journal of Australia 1: 5–11

Flynn M D, Edmonds M E, Tooke J E, Watkins P J 1988 Direct measurement of capillary blood flow in the diabetic neuropathic foot. Diabetologia 31: 652–656

Fuller R H, Shipley M J, Rose G, Jarrett R J, Keen H 1980 Coronary heart disease risk and impaired glucose tolerance. Lancet 1: 1373–1376

Ganda O P 1980 Pathogenesis of macrovascular disease in the human diabetic. Diabetes 29: 931–942

Goldenberg S, Alex M, Joshi R A, Blumenthal H 1959 Non-atheromatous peripheral vascular disease of the lower extremity in diabetes mellitus. Diabetes 8: 261–273

Gordon T, Castelli S P, Hjortland M C, Kannell W B, Dawber T R 1977 High-density lipoprotein as a protective factor against coronary heart disease: the Framingham study. American Journal of Medicine 62: 707–714

Jarrett R J 1988 Is insulin atherogenic? Diabetologia 31: 71–75

Jarrett R J, McCartney P, Keen H 1982 The Bedford Survey: ten-year mortality rates in newly diagnosed diabetics, borderline diabetics and normoglycaemic controls and risk indices for coronary heart disease in borderline diabetics. Diabetologia 22: 79–84

Jones R L, Peterson C M 1981 The fluid phase of coagulation and the accelerated atherosclerosis of diabetes mellitus. Diabetes 30 (suppl 2): 33–38

Kannel W B, McGee D L 1979 Diabetes and cardiovascular risk factors: the Framingham study. Circulation 59: 8–13

Kastrup J, Lassen N A, Parving H-H 1984 Diabetic microangiopathy, a factor enhancing the functional significance of peripheral occlusive arteriosclerotic occlusive disease. Clinical Physiology 4: 367–369

Kastrup J, Norgaard T, Parving H-H, Lassen N A 1987 Decreased distensibility of resistance vessels of the skin in type 1 (insulin-dependent) diabetic patients with microangiopathy. Clinical Science 72: 123–130

Kastrup J, Norgaard T, Parving H-H, Henriksen O, Lassen N A 1985 Impaired autoregulation of blood flow in subcutaneous tissue of long-term type 1 (insulin-dependent) diabetic patients with microangiopathy: an index of arteriolar dysfunction. Diabetologia 28: 711–717

Keen H 1985 Prevalence of small vessel and large vessel disease in diabetic patients from 14 centres. The World Health Organization Multinational Study of Vascular Disease in Diabetics. Diabetologia 28 (suppl): 615–640

Keen H, Jarrett R J, Fuller J H, McCartney P 1981 Hyperglycemia and arterial disease. Diabetes 30 (suppl 2): 49–53

Koenig R J, Cerami A 1980 Haemoglobin A_{IC} and diabetes mellitus. Annual Review of Medicine 31: 29–34

Ledet T 1981 Diabetic macroangiopathy and growth hormone. Diabetes 30 (suppl 2): 14–17

LoGerfo F W, Coffman J D 1984 Vascular and microvascular disease of the foot in diabetes, implications for foot care. New England Journal of Medicine 311: 1615–1619

Marinelli M R, Beach K W, Glass M J, Primozich J F, Strandness D E 1979 Non-invasive testing vs clinical evaluation of arterial disease. Journal of the American Medical Association 241: 2031–2034

Masarei J R L, Kiiveri H T, Stanton K 1986 Risk factors for cardiovascular disease in a diabetic population. Pathology 18: 89–93

Moore J M, Frew I D O 1965 Peripheral vascular lesions in diabetes mellitus. British Medical Journal 2: 19–23

National Diabetes Data Group 1979 Classification and diagnosis of diabetes mellitus and other categories of glucose intolerance. Diabetes 28: 1039–1057

Neilubowicz J, Borkowski M, Baraniewski H 1975 Opening of arteriovenous anastomoses and trophic ulcer formation after peripheral nerve injury. Journal of Cardiovascular Surgery 48: 100–115

Neubauer B 1971 A quantitative study of peripheral arterial calcification and glucose tolerance in elderly diabetics and non-diabetics. Diabetologia 7: 409–413

Nielsen P E 1973 Does diabetic microangiopathy cause development of gangrene? Scandinavian Journal of Clinical and Laboratory Investigation 31 (suppl 128): 229–234

Partsh H 1977 Neuropathies of the ulcero-mutilating types — clinical aspects, classification, circulation measurements. Vasa (suppl) 6: 1–48

Parving H H 1976 Increased microvascular permeability to plasma proteins in short- and long-term juvenile diabetics. Diabetes 25 (suppl 2): 884–889

Parving H H, Kastrup J, Smidt U M 1985 Reduced transcapillary escape of albumin during acute blood pressure lowering in Type 1 (insulin-dependent) diabetic patients with nephropathy. Diabetologia 28: 797–801

Rayman G, Hassan A, Tooke J E 1986 Blood flow in the skin of the foot related to posture in diabetes mellitus. British Medical Journal 292: 87–90

Reckless J P D, Betteridge D J, Wu P, Payne B, Galton D J 1978 High-density and low-density lipoproteins and prevalence of vascular disease in diabetes mellitus. British Medical Journal 1: 883–886

Robertson E B, Strong J P 1968 Atherosclerosis in persons with hypertension and diabetes mellitus. Laboratory Investigation 18: 538–551

Ross R 1986 The pathogenesis of atherosclerosis — an update. New England Journal of Medicine 314: 488–500.

Stary H C 1966 Disease of small blood vessels in diabetes mellitus. American Journal of the Medical Sciences 252: 357–374

Stolar M W 1988 Atherosclerosis in diabetes: the role of hyperinsulinaemia. Metabolism 37 (suppl 1): 1–9

Stout R W 1981 The role of insulin in atherosclerosis in diabetics and non-diabetics, a review. Diabetes 30 (suppl 2): 54–57

Strandness D E, Priest R E, Gibbons G E 1964 Combined clinical and pathologic study of diabetic and non-diabetic peripheral arterial disease. Diabetes 13: 366–372

Suarez L, Barrett-Connor E 1984 Interaction between cigarette smoking and diabetes mellitus in the prediction of death attributed to cardiovascular disease. American Journal of Epidemiology 120: 670–675

Tooke J E 1980 A capillary pressure disturbance in young diabetics. Diabetes 29: 815–819

Tooke J E 1986 Microvascular haemodynamics in diabetes mellitus. Clinical Science 70: 119–125

Vaccaro O, Pauciullo P, Rubba P et al 1985 Peripheral arterial circulation in individuals with impaired glucose tolerance. Diabetes Care 8/6: 594–597

Vague P, Juhan I 1983 Red cell deformability, platelet aggregation, and insulin action. Diabetes 32 (suppl 2 pt 2): 88–91

Vracko R 1970 Skeletal muscle capillaries in diabetics. Circulation 41: 271–283

Wahlberg F 1966 Intravenous glucose tolerance in myocardial infarction, angina pectoris and intermittent claudication. Acta Medica Scandanavica 180 (suppl 453): 1–93

Ward J D, Simms J M, Knight G, Boulton A J M, Sandler D A 1983 Venous distension in the diabetic neuropathic foot (physical sign of arteriovenous shunting). Journal of the Royal Society of Medicine 76: 1011–1014

West K M 1978 Epidemiology of diabetes and its vascular lesions. Elsevier, New York, ch 10

West K M et al 1983 The role of circulating glucose and triglyceride concentrations and their interactions with other 'risk factors' as determinants of arterial disease in nine diabetic population samples from the WHO multinational study: Diabetes Care 6: 361–369

Williamson J R, Kilo C 1979 A common-sense approach resolves the basement membrane controversy in the NIH Pima Indian study. Diabetologia 17: 129–131

Williamson J R, Kilo C 1983 Capillary basement membranes in diabetes. Diabetes 32 (suppl 2): 96–100

4. Neuropathy

Pamela M. Le Quesne, Nicholas Parkhouse, Irwin Faris

INTRODUCTION

Impairment of nerve function is an important and frequent complication of diabetes. All types of fibres are involved so that motor, sensory and autonomic functions are affected. Minor degrees of impairment can be detected clinically in about one third of adult diabetics although quantitative electrophysiological and functional tests will be abnormal in a greater number of patients. The changes in nerve function may be detectable at the time of diagnosis of the diabetes and tend to be gradually progressive, although improvement can occur with good diabetic control and more rapid deterioration may follow periods when the diabetes has been poorly controlled.

Neuropathy is an important cause of symptoms in many patients but in others it may be asymptomatic and hence, unrecognized. Ignorance of the neuropathy does not protect the patient from complications and this is particularly important in the foot; patients with impaired nerve function in the foot are at risk of the complications of neuropathy whether or not they are aware of its presence. Neuropathy remains one of the major factors leading to the development of foot lesions in diabetics (see Ch. 2).

CLASSIFICATION AND EPIDEMIOLOGY

A variety of different types of neuropathy occur in diabetes. The first classification proposed by Leyden in 1893 distinguished neuralgic, paralytic and ataxic types of neuropathy (Dyck et al 1987). Subsequent classifications have attempted to include the distribution and type of nerve fibre involved and pathogenic mechanisms such as ischaemia or entrapment.

Autonomic neuropathy was recognized by Buzzard (1890), and is found in association with both symmetrical polyneuropathies and asymmetrical, proximal motor neuropathies.

Dyck et al (1987) emphasize the difficulty of a rigid classification and propose the following scheme based on anatomic distribution and symmetry, and associated pathology:

1. Symmetric distal polyneuropathy; encompassing sensory, autonomic and motor involvement
2. Symmetric proximal neuropathy
3. Asymmetric neuropathy (more than 25% difference between sides)
   a. Cranial
   b. Trunk-radiculopathy or mononeuropathy
   c. Limb plexus or mononeuropathy
   d. Multiple mononeuropathy
   e. Entrapment neuropathy
   f. Ischaemic nerve injury from acute arterial occlusion.

Symmetric distal polyneuropathy is unquestionably the most common form of diabetic neuropathy. The reported incidence of neuropathy in diabetic populations has varied from 0–93% (Thomas & Eliasson 1984) due partly to variations in the criteria for diagnosis of neuropathy and the sensitivity of methods used for detection of abnormality. Pirart (1978) found the prevalence of neuropathy by clinical examination alone to be 8% at the time of diagnosis rising at a linear rate with the duration of diabetes to 50% after 25 years.

CLINICAL FEATURES

The symptoms and signs of diabetic neuropathy reflect a variable combination of sensory, motor and autonomic nerve fibre abnormalities. The following quotation from Colby (1965) illustrates the diversity of features:

There is no diabetic neurologic syndrome, but rather a heterogeneous array of mononeuropathies, polyneuropathies, myelopathies and possibly encephalopathies, which vary in type, nature of onset, relationship to diabetic control, severity, prognosis and susceptibility to various therapeutic programmes. The vagaries of diabetic neurologic disorders are so numerous that their recital leads to discouraging confusion.

In the common distal symmetrical polyneuropathy, the sensory disturbance has a distal, glove and stocking distribution and sensation in the foot may be symptomatically reduced or absent. Sensory symptoms range from mild numbness of the toes to profound anaesthesia. Vibration perception and proprioception in the limbs are often disturbed and ankle jerks reduced or absent with mild distal muscle weakness. Spontaneous pains, dysaesthesias and paraesthesias are common associated symptoms. A variety of different kinds of pain may occur ranging from mild discomfort to severe lancinating or burning pain. Certain patients have contact paraesthesia or dysaesthesia and in a few there is cutaneous hypersensitivity indistinguishable from causalgia. Some individuals complain of spontaneous cutaneous burning pain, others of a relentless deep-seated bony pain. Spontaneous pain may be present with varying degrees of sensory impairment, including the impairment of pain perception to noxious stimuli.

Table 4.1   Manifestations of autonomic neuropathy

1. Heart (Ewing & Clarke 1986)
   a. Raised resting heart rate
   b. Postural hypotension
   c. Lack of beat-to-beat heart rate variation
   d. Abnormal baroreceptor responses (Bennett et al 1980)
   e. Painless myocardial infarction

2. Peripheral circulation and thermoregulation
   a. Abnormal vasomotor changes to:
      (i) vasoactive drugs
      (ii) temperature change
   b. Abnormalities of sweating

3. Gastrointestinal (Scarpello & Sladen 1978)
   a. Oesophagus — decreased strength of peristaltic contraction and decreased lower
      oesophageal sphincter tone (Hollis et al 1977)
   b. Stomach — delayed gastric emptying and reduced incidence of peptic ulcer
      (Baron 1974), reduced gastric acid output (Hosking et al 1975)
   c. Gallbladder atony (Grodzki et al 1968)
   d. Diarrhoea

4. Genitourinary system (Annals of Internal Medicine 1980)
   a. Loss of bladder sensation
   b. Impotence (Carlin 1988)
   c. Failure of ejaculation
   d. Loss of testicular sensation (Campbell et al 1974)

5. Others
   a. Pupillary changes (Smith et al 1978)
   b. Cardiorespiratory arrest
   c. Loss of awareness of hypoglycaemia

One type of severely painful neuropathy is of acute onset, often early in the course of the disease and associated with marked weight loss but little objective sensory impairment. The pain in this type of neuropathy improves with adequate diabetic control (Archer et al 1984).

Autonomic dysfunction may cause orthostatic hypotension with oedema, sweating disorder, gastroparesis, diarrhoea, bladder dysfunction and impotence. A fuller list of the consequences of autonomic neuropathy is shown in Table 4.1.

Autonomic neuropathy is frequently asymptomatic and objective testing has shown that its incidence parallels that of somatic neuropathy. In general autonomic neuropathy occurs at the same time as somatic neuropathy and pure sensorimotor or autonomic neuropathy is unusual. Peripheral circulatory disturbance and sweating disturbance in the foot due to autonomic neuropathy have been considered to play an important role in the development of diabetic foot complications and this is discussed further below.

PATHOLOGY

The predominant feature of diabetic polyneuropathy is nerve fibre loss especially in the nerves of the feet and legs, as noted at postmortem (Pryce 1893). This was variably interpreted as evidence for 'peripheral neuritis' (Buzzard 1890, Woltman & Wilder 1929) or axonal degeneration (Williamson 1904).

The finding of segmental demyelination in diabetic nerves (Thomas & Lascelles 1965) and hypertrophy of Schwann cells and perineural fibroblasts (Ballin & Thomas 1968) raised the possibility of a primary disease of Schwann cells resulting in demyelination and remyelination. Present evidence is in favour of an independent effect of diabetes on axons and Schwann cells (Thomas & Eliasson 1984). Quantitative postmortem studies have shown multifocal nerve fibre loss at the level of the segmental nerves, becoming more marked distally. Sugimura & Dyck (1982) have emphasised the proximal, multifocal loss of fibres which would be expected to summate to produce symmetrical distal neuropathy. The evidence from these studies favours the ischaemic aetiology of neuropathy discussed below.

Loss of unmyelinated fibres has been demonstrated in somatic and autonomic nerves by silver staining (Martin 1953a) and by electron microscopy (Behse et al 1977). An associated increase in the number of very small unmyelinated axons reported in cases of painful neuropathy (Brown et al 1976) may indicate concurrent axonal regeneration with sprouting.

AETIOLOGY

In the past, nerve fibre damage was attributed to arteriosclerosis of the vasa nervorum. Woltman & Wilder (1929) found such changes in nerves taken from amputated gangrenous limbs and at postmortem of diabetic patients. However, in their study, normal neural structures of unknown genesis known as Renaut bodies were confused with infarcts (Sugimura & Dyck 1982). Furthermore, diabetic polyneuropathy is found in patients who exhibit no signs of major peripheral vascular disease (Downie & Newell 1961).

A more recent view is that hyperglycaemia and the consequent metabolic derangements may play an important part in the development of diabetic neuropathy. Neuropathy has been correlated with poor diabetic control and several studies have shown either improvement or lack of expected deterioration in various aspects of nerve function with careful diabetic control (usually using continuous subcutaneous insulin infusion) compared with conventional treatment (Holman et al 1983, Service et al 1985, Jakobsen et al 1988). Nevertheless, there is increasing evidence for a vascular component to the aetiology of diabetic peripheral neuropathy.

Metabolic abnormality

Hyperglycaemia causes a variety of metabolic abnormalities which might directly affect neural tissue:

1. Sorbitol and fructose accumulation (Gabbay 1975)
2. Intraneural myoinositol deficiency (Greene et al 1975)
3. Reduced Na^+/K^+ ATPase activity (Das et al 1976)
4. Non-enzymatic glycosylation of nerve proteins (Vlassara et al 1981, Brownlee et al 1988)
5. Impaired axoplasmic transport (Sidenius & Jakobsen 1982).

The increased activity of the polyol pathway due to hyperglycaemia results in accumulation of sorbitol and fructose which has metabolic and osmotic effects. These changes have been summarized by Asbury (1988) and a leading article in the Lancet (1989). Specific aldose reductase inhibitors which prevent the accumulation of sorbitol, improve conduction velocity in streptozotocin diabetic rats (Yue et al 1982). But as yet there is no positive consensus from clinical trials that either myoinositol supplements or aldose reductase inhibitors reverse the changes of human diabetic neuropathy (Judzewitsch et al 1983, Fagius et al 1985).

The conduction slowing and resistance of nerves to acute ischaemia in experimental diabetes in the rat is unaccompanied by histological changes and may be more amenable to biochemical manipulation than the chronic structural changes of established neuropathy in humans.

Ischaemia: diabetic vascular disease

Vascular changes affecting large and small vessels may contribute to peripheral nerve disease.

Large vessel disease

The arteriosclerosis that occurs in major vessels in diabetes differs from that in non-diabetics in its increased incidence, accelerated progress and more distal distribution.

Diabetic microangiopathy

The major features of diabetic microangiopathy are discussed in Chapter 3 and include increased capillary permeability and increased thickness of basement membranes. The endothelium becomes hyperpermeable to a range of molecules from small ions to albumin. Increased micropinocytosis of glycosylated albumin and its deposition on the basement membrane may contribute to its thickening. The altered basement membrane may then itself become more permeable. A permeability disorder at the blood-perineurial barrier could lead to endoneurial metabolic derangements and thence to neuropathy.

Intraluminal changes have been reported in capillaries within the endoneurium. Fagerberg (1959) described endothelial thickening and hyalinization of the small vessels in a large series of sural nerve biopsies from patients with diabetic neuropathy. In a later study, Timperley et al (1976) examined 24 sural nerve biopsies from diabetic patients with symptomatic neuropathy and reduced conduction velocity. In 9 cases thrombosis of endoneural vessels was found to be associated with focal areas of necrosis in the nerve fibres. In a further study of 11 sural nerve biopsies from patients with severe motor neuropathy, electron microscopy showed endothelial hyperplasia in all cases and plugging of the vascular lumen in seven patients (Timperley et al 1985). Postmortem morphometric studies in patients with diabetic polyneuropathy have demonstrated multifocal lesions in proximal nerve trunks presumed to summate to produce the symmetrical distal deficit (Dyck et al 1986, Johnson et al 1986).

Although some of the above studies have been criticised on the grounds that they looked mainly at elderly diabetic subjects, they do provide increasing evidence for a vascular component in the aetiology of diabetic neuropathy. However, there must still be reservations about accepting microvascular disease as the sole cause of diabetic neuropathy (Thomas 1987) and the relative contribution of the various suggested aetiological factors is still unknown (Asbury 1988, Lancet 1989).

METHODS OF ASSESSMENT AND FINDINGS

Peripheral nerves are composed of a mixture of fibres which may be distinguished morphologically and functionally (Table 4.2). They have been divided into groups according to fibre size and conduction velocity. Aγ fibres are the largest diameter and fastest conducting myelinated fibres and Aδ the smallest and slowest of the myelinated fibres. C fibres are unmyelinated and conduct much more slowly than myelinated fibres. Sensory nerve studies in primates and microneurographic studies in conscious man have defined the fibre groups responsible for different sensory modalities (Vallbo et al 1979).

In many types of peripheral neuropathy the largest diameter and longest nerve fibres are damaged most severely. This produces the typical clinical syndrome of distal glove and stocking sensory disturbances, particularly of vibration and proprioception sensation and weakness of the extremities, the lower limbs being affected more than the upper limbs because of their greater length. This picture, common to many metabolic and toxic conditions, has been termed a 'dying back' process or more recently a peripheral distal axonopathy (Spencer & Schaumburg 1976). The vulnerability of the largest and longest fibres is attributed to the greater cellular mass supported by the neurone.

It has long been known that the pattern described above does not apply to diabetic neuropathy. Clinical and pathological evidence has indicated that small diameter nerve fibres are vulnerable in this disease (Behse et al 1977,

Table 4.2 Functions and conduction velocities of peripheral nerve fibres. Ranges of conduction velocities approximate, detailed data not available for human nerves

	Aγβ (30–65 m/s)	Aα (15–40 m/s)	Aδ (5–20 m/s)	C (0.5–2 m/s)
Motor	Extrafusal	Intrafusal		
Muscle sensory	Muscle spindle Golgi tendon		Nociceptors	Nociceptors
Cutaneous sensory	Mechanoreceptor touch vibration pressure		Cool receptor Nociceptors (high threshold mechanoreceptors)	Warm receptor Polymodal nocicept
Autonomic				Sudomotor Vasomotor

Said et al 1983, Brown & Asbury 1984). The incidence of autonomic neuropathy, affecting peripheral unmyelinated C fibres, has already been discussed. Now with the advent of electrophysiological, psychophysical and functional tests it is possible to quantify the abnormalities in specific nerve fibre groups. Many studies have been concerned with determining the differential vulnerability of different types of peripheral nerve fibre in various clinical types of diabetic neuropathy (Guy et al 1985, Heimans et al 1986, Levy et al 1987, Ziegler et al 1988, Le Quesne et al 1990).

This type of study is important for three main reasons. Determination of the most sensitive test for detecting neuropathy is important in epidemiological studies. With the advent of potential new treatments, such as the aldose reductase inhibitors, it is important to be able to detect objectively whether there has been improvement or deterioration in nerve function. Determining whether there are particular patterns of nerve involvement in different clinical syndromes, such as the various foot disorders, may provide clues to their aetiology and hence pointers to preventive measures.

Electrophysiology

The mainstay of quantitative assessment of peripheral nerve function has for many years depended on electrophysiological measurement. Large diameter nerve fibres are stimulated and either the muscle or the compound sensory action potential is recorded. Nerve conduction velocity is frequently abnormal.

The amplitude of the evoked muscle action potential recorded through surface electrodes gives an indication of the number of functional motor units. Le Quesne & Fowler (1986) found a reduction in amplitude of the evoked potential from the flexor hallucis in the foot in patients with diabetic neuropathy, recorded following stimulation of the posterior tibial nerve.

The sural nerve is the most accessible sensory nerve for examination in the lower limb. In severe neuropathy and in some elderly subjects no potential may be recordable but when present the amplitude of the potential gives a useful measure of the number of surviving large diameter nerve fibres. In several studies where different groups of nerve fibres have been quantified, amplitude of sensory nerve action potentials has been found to be among the most frequently abnormal measure (Levy et al 1987, Guy et al 1988, Le Quesne et al 1990).

Quantitative sensory testing

Many small myelinated and unmyelinated fibres are not assessed by electrophysiological techniques. For the reasons discussed above the recently introduced techniques of quantitative sensory testing (Dyck et al 1984) have been increasingly used in the study of diabetic neuropathy. These techniques have been made possible by the incorporation of graded and modality-specific stimuli in psychophysical tests for the different nerve fibre groups recognized physiologically (Lindblom 1981).

Aβ mechanosensitive fibres

The integrity of these fibres may be assessed by measuring the threshold for appreciation of vibration sensation. Various methods have been described, for example Dyck et al (1984) employed precisely controlled amplitudes of vibration as stimuli and asked the patient to choose which of two test periods contained the stimulus (forced choice). Stimulus strength is varied according to the response and threshold determined, applying a protocol which embodies established psychophysical principles.

The Biothesiometer (Ohio) is a commonly used and less elaborate device which compares well with other instruments (Salle & Verberck 1984). The technique is simple. A probe is placed on the skin, the amplitude of vibration of which can be controlled. Threshold is taken as the stimulus amplitude at which sensation is felt as amplitude is increased or disappears as amplitude is reduced (psychophysical method of limits). The results are reproducible and sensitive, detecting the change in threshold to be expected with increasing age (Bloom et al 1984, Le Quesne & Fowler 1987). The instrument is widely used by diabetologists. However, some calibration of the commercially available machine is necessary (Le Quesne et al 1990).

Vibration perception threshold is a good functional measure of the integrity of one group of large myelinated sensory fibres. It is often abnormal, particularly when neuropathy is advanced (Le Quesne et al 1990), although in a number of studies it has been found abnormal slightly less frequently than thermal perception threshold (Guy et al 1985, Heimans et al 1986, Levy et al 1987, Ziegler et al 1988). It is a particularly useful measure for following the progress of the disease.

Aδ and C Fibres concerned with temperature sensation

Impulses induced by cooling stimuli are conducted in different fibres (Aδ) from those concerned with the sensation of warmth (C fibres). Various devices have been evolved to measure thermal appreciation threshold. In modern times a Peltier device is used consisting of two dissimilar metals in contact. The temperature of the device changes when a current is passed, the direction of change depending on the direction of current. The Marstock device measures the difference between warm and cold appreciation (Fruhstorfer et al 1976) which has been found to be sensitive for the detection of diabetic neuropathy (Navarro et al 1989). In other systems, cooling and warming thresholds are measured separately, thus giving information about Aδ and C fibres independently (Fowler et al 1987). Warming threshold is usually found to be the more abnormal (Fowler et al 1987, Sosenko et al 1988, Le Quesne et al 1990).

Measurement of thermal threshold has proved a valuable technique for detection of disorders of small diameter somatic peripheral nerves. The high incidence of abnormal thermal perception, and warming in particular, provides clear evidence that small diameter nerve fibres are frequently involved in diabetic neuropathy. However, none of the studies mentioned has shown clear evidence of selective damage to small fibres. A few patients with mild clinical neuropathy may show defects confined to small fibres (Le Quesne et al 1990) but all fibre groups become involved as neuropathy becomes more severe.

Nociceptive fibres

Pain sensation is subserved by two groups of nerve fibres: the rapidly conducting, high-threshold mechanosensitive myelinated Aδ fibres responsible for sharp, 'first' pain and the polymodal nonmyelinated nociceptive C fibres responsible for dull, burning pain. Many methods for measurement of the function of fibres concerned with the sensation of pain have depended on subjective assessment and thus are open to many modulating influences. A variety of types of stimulation have been used to determine the threshold for pain appreciation. Although valuable information has been obtained about various aspects of pain appreciation in normal subjects using elaborate psychophysical testing procedures, these techniques have been difficult to apply to clinical problems.

Le Quesne & Fowler (1986) measured pinch pain threshold quantitatively on the dorsum of the foot with a pinchometer (Lynn & Perl 1977). In control subjects the first change in sensation was a sharp pain similar to the descriptions of 'first pain', and presumably dependent on stimulation of Aδ fibres. In diabetic subjects the main abnormality was not an increase in threshold but an increased variability in threshold at different sites on the dorsum of the foot. In a proportion of the diabetic subjects pain was not appreciated at one or more points when the maximum force (2.8 kg) was used. In other subjects the quality of pain was altered; in some a dull ache (presumably related to nociceptive C fibre activity) rather than a sharp pain (related to Aδ activity) was felt; in others pain was referred to a site other than that stimulated and in some, pain was appreciated at an abnormally low level of stimulation. The loss of sharp pain appreciation and abnormal quality of pain produced was interpreted as being due to loss of Aδ fibres, and the low threshold response was thought to be due to stimulation of collateral sprouts of surviving fibres or the abnormally sensitive tips of regenerating fibres. Thus, this method gave better qualitative than quantitative information about disturbed pain appreciation.

Various other methods have been used clinically for the assessment of nociceptive C fibres, such as the pain threshold to intense heating. Heat pain is a function of polymodal nociceptive C fibres and not the C fibres responsible for the sensation of warming. Like warming threshold it can be measured using the Marstock apparatus.

However, nociceptive C fibres have a dual role. Not only do they transmit afferent impulses to the central nervous system, where they are interpreted as pain, but they are also concerned with the initiation of neurogenic inflammation, via an axon reflex. This local reflex causes the spreading flare, the properties of which were delineated by Sir Thomas Lewis (1927). Impulses travel centrally from a site of injury to the skin and then pass to an efferent branch where they terminate in relation to mast cells and cutaneous microvessels. Vasodilatation results from the release of histamine and neuropeptides, particularly substance P (Foreman 1987).

Capitalizing on the dual function of nociceptive C fibres, Parkhouse & Le Quesne (1988a) have developed a more objective technique for quantifying them by measuring the flare. An axon reflex is stimulated by electrophoresis of acetylcholine and its intensity is measured with a laser Doppler flowmeter. These authors found a reduced or absent flare in diabetics, particularly those with foot complications (vide infra).

An abnormal histamine flare has previously been described in diabetes (Starr 1930) but often attributed to vascular rather than neural disease. Previous authors (eg Hutchison et al 1974, Aronin et al 1987) have not considered the implications of a reduced flare indicating a reduction in the neurogenic inflammatory response to injury.

Autonomic system

Stimulation of peripheral sympathetic nerves to the limbs causes vasoconstriction and sweating. The autonomic system is also involved in a number of cardiac and vascular reflexes.

Peripheral vasomotor system

Abnormalities of the neural control of the vessels in the limbs were among the first manifestations of autonomic neuropathy to be studied. The limb vessels have an important role in regulation of body temperature in addition to their function in perfusing the tissues of the limb.

A number of authors have demonstrated a reduced vasodilator response to body heating and reduced responses following the injection of vasoactive drugs. These changes were initially attributed to the presence of small vessel disease and the tests were advocated for its diagnosis, but a more likely explanation for the findings has been given by Moorhouse et al (1966) who studied the responses of the peripheral circulation to changes in temperature. They found that in subjects with chronic sympathetic denervation, as occurs in diabetics, the reflex responses related to requirements of internal temperature homeostasis did not occur. Instead, the vessels exhibited a local autonomy which was dependent on local temperature. Thus, vessels which did not dilate in response to heating the trunk would dilate if the limb was immersed in warm water. In addition the vasoconstriction which followed immersion of the foot in cold water was intense and prolonged.

More direct methods have become available recently for studying the peripheral vasomotor system. Microneurography in humans has confirmed that sympathetic neural discharges in skin nerves are associated with the manoeuvres that are recognized to cause vasoconstriction eg startle, inspiratory gasp and cold stimuli to a remote part of the body (Vallbo et al 1979). In some diabetic patients the absence of discharges in response to such stimuli indicates peripheral vasomotor denervation (Fagius 1982). However, microneurographic studies do not easily give a quantitative estimate of partial denervation.

In 1983, Low et al (1983a) described the use of a laser Doppler flow meter for measuring changes in skin blood flow following sympathetic activating stimuli and demonstrated diminished or absent responses in some neuropathic patients. Using a similar technique, Le Quesne et al (1990) found the incidence of absent responses on the sole of the foot increased with the clinical severity of somatic neuropathy.

However, detailed quantitative assessment of disturbed peripheral vasomotor innervation is still not possible.

Sweating

Pryce (1893) first described alteration of sweating in diabetic neuropathy. In past clinical studies, the presence or absence of sweating has often been determined by assessing the colour change following topical application of either starch and iodine, or quinizarine powder that changes colour when moist (Barany & Cooper 1956). More recently, the psychogalvanic response of the skin has been recorded as an indirect measure of sweating. This response was found to be abnormal more frequently in patients with foot ulcers than in those without (Deanfield et al 1980).

Direct measurement of sweat production on the dorsum of the foot has been achieved in several studies. Kennedy et al (1984a) measured the number of active glands and the volume of sweat produced from the impression of the sweat droplets in silastic dental impression material. Sweating was stimulated locally by electrophoresis of pilocarpine, to which denervated sweat glands do not respond (an exception to Cannon's law of denervation hypersensitivity). The magnitude of the defect in sweating was measured in diabetics with varying degrees of neuropathy (Kennedy et al 1984a,b).

Low et al (1983b) described the Quantitative Sudomotor Axon Reflex Test (QSART) dependent on measurement of sweat produced by an axon reflex stimulated by electrophoresis of acetylcholine into the skin. Using this technique, Ahmed & Le Quesne (1986) found that sweating was absent on the dorsum of foot in 27, and reduced in 7, of 52 diabetic feet.

In contrast to the common finding of deficient sweating, excessive sweat production can occur in certain circumstances in diabetes. Diabetic patients sometimes experience a period when they sweat excessively on their feet before losing the ability to sweat completely. The explanation for this is unknown. It could possibly be similar to the hyperaesthesiae which are a common manifestation of somatic neuropathy, i.e. spontaneous or excess discharges in response to stimuli in partially damaged fibres.

Hyperhydrosis of the upper part of the body may occur in patients who have lost the capacity to sweat distally and is probably a compensatory mechanism. Abnormal sweating of the face after eating (Watkins 1973) is probably due to local nerve abnormality (auriculotemporal nerve) rather than necessarily being part of a widespread change.

Cardiovascular autonomic reflexes

These reflexes have been intensively studied and the subject has been reviewed by Ewing & Clarke (1986). The detection of changes may be of prognostic importance. In a small series (Ewing et al 1976) more than half the patients with symptomatic autonomic neuropathy and abnormal cardiovascular reflexes died within $2\frac{1}{2}$ years. This does not mean that the deaths were due to autonomic neuropathy although there are several mechanisms by which the effects of autonomic neuropathy might lead to death, e.g. cardiac arrhythmias, unawareness of hypoglycaemia and abnormalities of the control of ventilation.

A battery of five simple tests has been proposed for the detection of cardiovascular autonomic dysfunction (Ewing et al 1985). Three of the tests measure heart rate responses to three different cardiovascular stimuli: deep breathing, standing up and the Valsalva manoeuvre. The other two measure blood pressure responses to standing up and to sustained handgrip.

Beat-to-beat variation in heart rate. The variation which occurs in heart rate in normal subjects is largely due to changes in vagal activity in response to afferent stimuli from pulmonary stretch receptors. This variation is reduced in autonomic neuropathy. It can be assessed in several

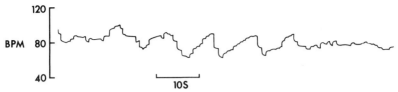

Fig. 4.1 Heart rate changes during deep breathing. Normal subject. There is an accentuation of the normal sinus arrythmia.

ways. (1) Maximal variation in heart rate can be induced by deep breathing at the rate of 6 breaths per minute. In normal subjects the rate varies by 15 or more beats per minute under this stimulus (Fig. 4.1). (2) The shorter stimulus of a single maximal inspiration followed by exhalation produces a transient fall in heart rate. The change is less in a patient with a denervated heart. (3) The standard deviation of the heart rate, measured over a specified period, e.g. 5 minutes, is large in normal subjects and small in those whose heart rate varies least.

Valsalva manoeuvre. This is the classic manoeuvre for studying autonomic reflexes affecting the circulation. Complete evaluation of the response requires arterial pressure monitoring (Fig. 4.2) but the heart rate changes provide a reliable guide to the circulatory changes (Fig. 4.3). The patient maintains an expiratory pressure of 30 mm mercury for 10–15 seconds. In normal subjects the heart rate increases during this period. Following relaxation, the heart rate continues to rise for a few beats and then a profound bradycardia develops. It is the reduction or absence of this bradycardia which is the characteristic finding in autonomic neuropathy.

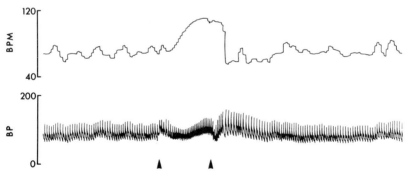

Fig. 4.2 Valsalva manoeuvre. Blood pressure and heart rate changes in a normal subject. There are several phases of the response.

1. An initial rise in blood pressure as the rise in intrathoracic pressure is transmitted to the great vessels.

2. A fall in blood pressure due to reduced venous filling of the heart. This results in a baroreflex-induced tachycardia with restoration of blood pressure.

3. When the pressure is released (second arrow) there is a sudden increase in filling of the heart. Cardiac output rises and so does the blood pressure ('overshoot'). This produces a bradycardia mediated via the baroreflexes.

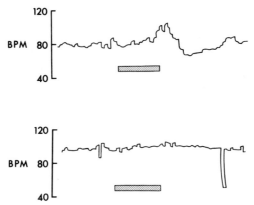

Fig. 4.3 Valsalva manouevre. Heart rate changes in a normal subject (above) and in a diabetic (below). In the diabetic the only change is a small increase in heart rate during the 10 s period of the stimulus (indicated by the shaded marker). Note the higher resting heart rate in the diabetic.

This test has the advantages of being simple, non-invasive and reproducible, and is within the capacity even of frail subjects.

Postural changes in blood pressure and heart rate. When one stands from a lying position there is pooling of blood in the legs which produces a fall in venous return and thus cardiac output. The normal compensatory responses are tachycardia and peripheral vasoconstriction both of which tend to maintain the normal blood pressure. In autonomic neuropathy there is a smaller rise in heart rate and, because there is reduced peripheral vasoconstriction, the blood pressure falls. Both the heart rate and blood pressure changes are easy to detect without arterial cannulation. An abnormal blood pressure response results in a fall of greater than 30 mm mercury.

Blood pressure response to isometric exercise. During isometric exercise the blood pressure and heart rate rise. The afferent stimuli arise from exercising muscles and the effector mechanisms involve a reduction in vagal tone on the heart and peripheral vasoconstriction. In response to a standard exercise (e.g. sustaining 30% of maximal voluntary contraction), a rise in diastolic blood pressure of less than 10 mm mercury is considered to be abnormal.

Table 4.3 summarizes the results of these tests.

Although the cardiovascular reflexes have been categorized as sympathetic or parasympathetic, Ewing et al (1984) have advocated a less clear distinction between these two systems with categorization of the abnormality as early, definite and severe. Heart rate responses are usually involved first, but it is unwise to rely on a single test for diagnosis or quantification. The use of only a single heart rate variability test probably accounted for the low incidence of abnormality found by Le Quesne et al (1990) in diabetics, including those with severe peripheral neuropathy.

A more sensitive technique for detecting cardiovascular autonomic dys-

Table 4.3 Bedside tests of autonomic function

	Normal	Borderline	Abnormal
Beat-to beat changes			
Max-min rate (bpm)	>15	11–14	<10
Standard deviation of RR interval (ms)	> 50		
Valsalva ratio	>1.20	1.11–1.20	<1.10
Postural change			
HR 30:15 ratio	>1.03	1.01–1.03	<1.00
Fall in diastolic BP	<10	11–29	>30
(mm Hg)			
Isometric exercise	>15	10–15	<10
Rise in diastolic BP			
(mm Hg)			

function, but of less practical application, is to determine whether there is a reduction in the sudden large changes in heart rate that occur frequently during the day and night in normal subjects (Ewing et al 1984). Twenty four-hour ECG monitoring is required.

Another common manifestation of diabetic autonomic neuropathy is impotence. Fowler et al (1988) found a close correlation in diabetics between abnormality of warming perception on the feet and neurogenic impotence, both dependent on unmyelinated C fibres.

In general, autonomic neuropathy deteriorates in proportion to somatic neuropathy (Ahmed et al 1986). However, Young et al (1986) concluded that 'different fibre types may be involved in varying proportions with the different clinical presentations'.

A number of studies incorporating a variety of nerve function tests have been discussed. These vary in detail but, not surprisingly, show a general deterioration of function with increased clinical severity of neuropathy and with the onset of complications. The majority of patients show diffuse involvement of all fibre groups, albeit to different degrees. The result of applying a battery of nerve function tests to various groups of diabetics is shown in Table 4.4.

It is important to stress that the incidence of abnormality of the various tests does not necessarily reflect the relative number of nerve fibres damaged. The sensitivity of the tests varies, due, among other factors, to the nature and design of the tests, to the biological variability in control subjects, and to the amount of summation necessary for conscious sensation. One of the reasons why warmth sensation is so frequently abnormal is that many nerve fibres need to be stimulated simultaneously (a high degree of summation) before a conscious sensation is produced. Hence the sensation is lost when only a few fibres degenerate. Nevertheless, in broad terms these tests give an indication of the relative involvement of different fibre groups and in practice it is possible to decide on suitable tests for screening for neuropathy and for following progress.

Table 4.4 Percentage of patients with abnormalities of various nerve functions

Fibre type			Aγb			Aδ	C				
							Somatic		Autonomic		
Group	n	Svel	Samp	Mamp	Vib	Cool	Warm	C noc	Sweat*	Vasom	Btdif
I	11	0	36	18	36	0	45	27	20	0	0
II	27	33	81	44	81	33	59				27
III	23	70	95	78	87	78	96	83	52	33	53

Group I: 11 patients with long-standing diabetes but clinically insignificant neuropathy
Group II: 27 patients with mild neuropathy
Group III: 23 patients with neuropathic foot lesions

SVEL = sural nerve conduction velocity; SAMP = sural nerve action potential amplitude; MAMP = adductor hallucis muscle action potential amplitude; VIB = vibration perception threshold; COOL = cooling perception threshold; WARM = warming perception threshold; C NOC = flare response; BTDIF = RR interval variability
* Sweating was absent on the soles of 20% of control subjects.
(From Le Quesne et al 1990, with permission)

NEUROPATHIC FOOT COMPLICATIONS

The first suggestion that plantar ulceration might be due to a neurological deficit was made by Duplay & Morat in 1873 and the association between plantar ulceration, neuropathy and vascular disease was made by Pryce (1887). Since that time neuropathy, particularly its sensory component, has been widely recognized as an important factor in the formation of the diabetic plantar ulcer, interacting with connective tissue changes (Delbridge et al 1985a) and mechanical forces (Stokes et al 1975, Delbridge et al 1985b).

The development of Charcot joints in patients with diabetes mellitus was first documented by Jordan (1936). It was generally regarded as rare until Martin (1953b) published his study of 150 patients with neuropathy in which 9 (6%) had neuropathic bone and joint lesions.

Sensory changes

The most significant abnormality in the development of foot lesions is the inability to perceive pain. This predisposes the foot to direct mechanical injury from treading on sharp objects, burning, and the repetitive mechanical forces of gait. The common feature in all these examples is failure to perceive the presence of a harmful agent, which in a normal person, would be noticed by the pain it caused and would be removed. Infection goes unnoticed and may progress to spreading cellulitis or deep abscess formation.

A characteristic of infection in the diabetic neuropathic foot is lack of erythema accompanying the lack of pain. In many cases, the lack of inflammatory response is at least partly due to neuropathy. Degeneration of nociceptive C fibres predisposes to foot lesions in two distinct ways: by impairment of protective pain sensation (the afferent component) and by impairment of the neurogenic inflammatory response to injury (the efferent component) (Parkhouse & Le Quesne 1988b).

Although Sir Thomas Lewis (1937) recognized the adaptive advantages of the dual function system, which he called the nocifensor system, the efferent function has been historically neglected in favour of the loss of pain sensation. It is, however, a clinical observation that denervated but otherwise normal tissue is slow to heal and is prone to cutaneous lesions and ulceration (Learmonth 1953). Wybauw (1938) observed increased oedema and necrosis at the site of inflammation in rabbits after sensory nerves were cut and allowed to degenerate. However, the clinical importance of neurogenic inflammation in the overall response to injury has not been fully elucidated. It seems possible that it may be at least as important as pain sensation.

Charcot (1868) emphasized the central importance of loss of pain sensation in the joint destruction which he originally described. Dysfunction of the nociceptor fibres may be the most prominent abnormality in an otherwise relatively normal neuropathic profile. For example, a twenty-year-old woman rapidly developed a florid Charcot foot after painless mild trauma. She had a markedly abnormal flare, but the only other neurogenic dysfunction to be detected was mild conduction slowing and impaired warmth perception.

Motor changes

Denervation of muscles has important effects on the function of the foot. The small muscles of the foot, the extensor digitorum brevis, lumbrical and interosseus muscles are commonly affected. The actions of these muscles are similar to those of the corresponding muscles in the hand. They modulate the function of the long flexor and extensor muscles whose muscle bellies are remote from the site at which their tendons insert. The results of paralysis of the small muscles in the foot are analogous to the changes produced by denervation of the small muscles of the hand, e.g. by division of the deep branch of the ulnar nerve. The metatarsophalangeal joints are hyperextended and the interphalangeal joints are flexed. The joints initially remain mobile but later degenerative changes occur and the joints become fixed.

The deformity produced by denervation predisposes to the development of ulcers. As the toes become clawed abnormal pressure may develop on the tips and occasionally ulcers form there (Fig. 8.8). More often trauma occurs to the dorsum of the flexed and dorsally displaced proximal interphalangeal joint. A similar deformity may occur in non-diabetics. It probably results from muscle weakness associated with ageing but, apart from callus formation over the flexed interphalangeal joint, seldom causes any serious difficulties for the patient. The reason for the difference between diabetic and non-diabetic is that the former has pain sensation in the area and thus small injuries are noticed and treated. In the diabetic with neuropathy, progressive tissue damage may occur.

Autonomic changes

In recent times it has been suggested that autonomic neuropathy contributes to the pathogenesis of ulceration, neuropathic oedema and Charcot arthropathy. Quantitative impairment of sweating and blood flow disturbance have both been measured in these conditions. Microneurographic recording suggests that sudomotor and skin vasoconstrictor functions may be impaired, sometimes independently (Fagius 1982).

Impairment of sweating is suggested to contribute, through dehydration, to the formation of hyperkeratotic plaques and fissures in the skin. The occurrence of similar changes in the anhydrous skin of neuropathic feet in leprosy suggests that this factor may be more important than abnormal glycosylation of keratin, which has been suggested as a contributory factor in diabetic ulceration (Delbridge et al 1985a). In a recent study, sympathetic sweating in response to acetylcholine electrophoresis was found to be reduced in most diabetics with neuropathic foot lesions but paradoxically increased in some diabetics with Charcot arthropathy (Ahmed & Le Quesne 1986). This observation highlights the differing nature of these two conditions, which are distinct clinically and probably in aetiology.

Sympathetic neuropathy may have important effects on the peripheral circulation producing vasodilatation due to diminished vascular tone and arteriovenous shunting (Edmonds et al 1982). These authors have suggested that the increased blood flow is responsible for demineralization and rarefaction of bone which in turn predisposes to recurrent, minor fractures resulting in Charcot arthropathy. In addition, arteriovenous shunting reduces the nutritional flow to the skin, predisposing the skin to ulceration, poor healing and sepsis (Ward et al 1983). The additional loss of the sympathetic veni-vasomotor postural reflex contributes, with the increased blood flow, to the formation of neuropathic oedema (Rayman et al 1986).

This concept is largely dependent on indirect evidence involving the measurement of pulse wave velocity and pulsatility indices calculated from ultrasound Doppler waveforms in the foot vessels (Edmonds et al 1982) and the finding of a reduced arteriovenous oxygen tension gradient (Boulton et al 1982). However, these changes could have been due to reduced arterial wall compliance in the absence of sympathetic dysfunction. And in one case, sympathetic vasoconstrictor reflexes were shown to be intact despite increased blood flow and decreased pulsatility indices (Archer et al 1984). However, there is direct evidence that arteriovenous shunting occurs, from the measurement of the transit of radiolabelled microspheres through the microcirculation.

Using a battery of cardiovascular autonomic function tests including postural hypotension and the heart rate responses to the Valsalva manoeuvre and deep breathing, Corbin et al (1987) found no clear association between autonomic neuropathy and the degree of abnormality of blood flow measured by Doppler waveform analysis in diabetic patients with and without symptomatic neuropathy and recurrent foot ulceration. More recently, peripheral sympathetic vasoconstrictor reflexes have been measured in the feet of diabetics with both ulceration and neuroarthropathy (Parkhouse & Le Quesne 1988b). The response was totally absent in only a small proportion of patients with foot complications. These discrepancies challenge the concept of a dominant role for circulatory disturbances due to sympathetic neuropathy in the pathogenesis of the various types of foot complication.

CONCLUSIONS

Diabetes remains the commonest cause of neuropathy in the Western world and is second only to leprosy as a cause worldwide. Intensive research is in progress to ellucidate the pathogenesis of the neuropathy. When this succeeds, definitive prophylactic measures should be available. In the meantime the best glycaemic control that can be achieved offers the most hopeful method of reducing the incidence of neuropathy and its attendent complications. Attempts at reversing metabolic derangements, e.g. with aldose reductase inhibitors, have not so far proved their clinical worth. This may be partly because of the length of time required to show an effect (possibly many years).

While the incidence of neuropathy remains high among diabetics, it remains important to try to understand the pathogenesis of the complications. A number of tests of varying degrees of complexity have been used in attempts to identify the functions that are most abnormal in diabetics with foot lesions. Certain tests, such as vibration perception threshold measured with a Biothesiometer, have proved clinically useful. However, it must be emphasized that most of the elaborate tests remain research tools at the present time. It is hoped that with increased understanding of the relative importance of the many contributory factors it will be possible to identify risk factors and to provide more specific prophylactic treatment.

REFERENCES

Annals of Internal Medicine 1980 92 (Part 2): 291–342
Ahmed M E, Delbridge L, Le Quesne L P 1986 The role of autonomic neuropathy in diabetic foot ulceration. Journal of Neurology, Neurosurgery and Psychiatry 49: 1002–1006

Ahmed M E, Le Quesne P M 1986 Quantitative sweat test in diabetics, with neuropathic foot lesions. Journal of Neurology, Neurosurgery and Psychiatry 49: 1059–1062

Archer A G, Roberts V C, Watkins P J 1984 Blood flow patterns in painful diabetic neuropathy. Diabetologia 27: 563–567

Aronin N, Leeman S E, Clements R E 1987 Diminished flare response in neuropathic diabetic patients. Diabetes 36: 1139–1143

Asbury A K 1988 Understanding diabetic neuropathy. New England Journal of Medicine 319: 577–578

Ballin R H M, Thomas P K 1968 Hypertrophic changes in diabetic neuropathy. Acta Neuropathologica 11: 93–102

Barany F R, Cooper E H 1956 Pilomotor and sudomotor innervation in diabetes. Clinical Science 15: 533–540

Baron J H 1974 Letter: Autonomic neuropathy and autovagotomy. British Medical Journal 3: 408–409

Behse F, Buchtal F, Carlsen F 1977 Nerve biopsy and conduction studies in diabetic neuropathy. Journal of Neurology, Neurosurgery and Psychiatry 40: 1072–1082

Bennett T, Hosking D J, Hampton J R 1980 Cardiovascular responses to graded reductions of central blood volume in normal subjects and in patients with diabetes mellitus. Clinical Science 58: 193–200

Bloom S, Till S, Sonsken P, Smith S 1984 Use of a biothesiometer to measure individual vibration thresholds and their variation in 519 non-diabetic subjects. British Medical Journal 288: 1793–1795

Boulton A J M, Scarpello J H B, Ward J D 1982 Venous oxygenation in the diabetic neuropathic foot: evidence of arteriovenous shunting? Diabetologia 22: 6–8

Brown M J, Asbury A K 1984 Diabetic neuropathy. Annals of Neurology 15: 2–12

Brown M J, Martin J R, Asbury A K 1976 Painful diabetic neuropathy. A morphometric study. Archives of Neurology 33: 164–171

Carlin B W 1988 Impotence and diabetes. Metabolism 37 (suppl 1): 19–21

Brownlee M, Cerami A, Vlassara H 1988 Advanced glycosylation end products in tissue and the biochemical basis of diabetic complications. New England Journal of Medicine 318: 1315–1321

Buzzard T 1890 Illustrations of some less known forms of peripheral neuritis, especially alcoholic monoplegia and diabetic neuritis. British Medical Journal 1: 1419–1422

Campbell I W, Ewing D J, Clarke B F, Duncan L J P 1974 Testicular pain sensation in diabetic autonomic neuropathy. British Medical Journal 2: 638–639

Charcot J M 1868 Sur quelques arthropathies qui paraissent dependre d'une lesion du cerveau ou de la moelle epiniere. Archives de Physiologie Normale et Pathologique 1: 161–168

Colby A O 1965 Neurologic disorders of diabetes mellitus. Diabetes 14: 424–429

Corbin D O C, Young R J, Morrison D C, Hoskins P, McDicken W N, Housley E, Clarke B F 1987 Blood flow in the foot, polyneuropathy and foot ulceration in diabetes mellitus. Diabetologia 30: 473–486

Das P K, Bray G M, Aguayo A J, Rasminsky M 1976 Diminished ouabain-sensitive sodium-potassium ATPase activity in sciatic nerves of rats with streptozotocin-induced diabetes. Experimental Neurology 53: 285–288

Deanfield J E, Daggett P R, Harrison M J G 1980 The role of autonomic neuropathy in diabetic foot ulceration. Journal of the Neurological Sciences 47: 203–210

Delbridge L, Ellis C S, Robertson K, Le Quesne L P 1985a Non-enzymatic glycosylation of keratin from the stratum corneum of the diabetic foot. British Journal of Dermatology 112: 547–554

Delbridge L, Ctercteko G, Fowler C, Reeve T S, Le Quesne L P 1985b The aetiology of diabetic neuropathic ulceration of the foot. British Journal of Surgery 72: 1–6

Downie A W, Newell D J 1961 Sensory nerve conduction in patients with diabetes mellitus and controls. Neurology 11: 876–882

Duplay S, Morat J P 1873 Recherches sur la pathogenie du mal perforant du pied (mal plantaire perforant). Archives generales de medecine March: 257–275

Dyck P J, Karnes J, O'Brien P C, Zimmerman I R 1984 Detection threshold of cutaneous sensation in humans. In: Dyck P J, Thomas P K, Lambert E H, Bunge R (eds) Peripheral neuropathy 2nd edn. W B Saunders, Philadelphia, p 1103–1138

Dyck P J, Karnes J L, O'Brien P, Okazaki H, Lais A, Engelstad J 1986 The spatial
distribution of fibre loss in diabetic polyneuropathy suggests ischaemia. Annals of
Neurology 19: 440–449

Dyck P J, Karnes J, O'Brien P C 1987 Diagnosis, staging and classification of diabetic
neuropathy and associations with other complications. In: Dyck P J, Thomas P K,
Asbury A K, Winegrad A I, Porte D (eds) Diabetic neuropathy. W B Saunders,
Philadelphia, p 36

Edmonds M E, Roberts V C, Watkins P J 1982 Blood flow in the diabetic neuropathic
foot. Diabetologia 22: 9–15

Ewing D J, Campbell I W, Clarke B F 1976 Mortality in diabetic autonomic neuropathy.
Lancet 1: 601–603

Ewing D J, Clarke B F 1986 Diabetic autonomic neuropathy: present insights and future
prospects. Diabetes Care 9: 648–665

Ewing D J, Martyn C N, Clarke B F 1985 The value of cardiovascular autonomic function
tests: 10 years experience in diabetes. Diabetes Care 8: 491–498

Ewing D J, Neilson J M M, Travis P 1984 New method for assessing cardiac
parasympathetic activity using 24-hour electrocardiograms. British Heart Journal
52: 396–402

Fagerberg S E 1959 Diabetic neuropathy, a clinical and histological study on the
significance of vascular affections. Acta Medica Scandinavica 164 (suppl 345): 1–80

Fagius J 1982 Microneurographic findings in diabetic polyneuropathy with special reference
to sympathetic nerve activity. Diabetologia 23: 415–420

Fagius J, Brattberg A, Jameson S, Berne C 1985 Limited benefit of treatment of diabetic
polyneuropathy with an aldose reductase inhibitor; a 24-week controlled trial.
Diabetologia 28: 323–329

Foreman J C 1987 Peptides and neurogenic inflammation. British Medical Bulletin
43: 386–400

Fowler C J, Ali Z, Kirby R S, Pryor J P 1988 The value of testing for unmyelinated fibre,
sensory neuropathy in diabetic impotence. British Journal of Urology 61: 63–67

Fowler C J, Carroll M C, Burns D, Howe N, Robinson K A 1987 A portable system for
measuring cutaneous thresholds for warmth and cold. Journal of Neurology,
Neurosurgery and Psychiatry 50: 1211–1215

Fruhstorfer H, Lindblom U, Schmidt W G 1976 Method for quantitative estimation of
thermal thresholds in patients. Journal of the neurological Sciences 39: 1071–1075

Gabbay K H 1975 Hyperglycaemia, polyol metabolism and complications of diabetes
mellitus. Annual Review of Medicine 26: 521–536

Greene D A, DeJesus P V, Winegrad A I 1975 Effects of insulin and dietary myoinositol
on impaired peripheral motor nerve conduction velocity in acute streptozotocin diabetes.
Journal of Clinical Investigation 55: 1326–1336

Grodzki M, Mazurkiewicz-Rozynska E, Czyzyk A 1968 Diabetic cholecystopathy.
Diabetologia 4: 345–348

Guy R J C, Clark C A, Malcolm P N, Watkins P J 1985 Evaluation of thermal and
vibration sensation in diabetic neuropathy. Diabetologia 28: 131–137

Guy R J C, Gilbey S G, Sheehy M, Asselman P, Watkins P J 1988 Diabetic neuropathy in
the upper limb and the effect of twelve months sorbinil treatment. Diabetologia
31: 214–220

Heimans J J, Bertelsmann F W, Van Rooy J C G M 1986 Large and small nerve fibre
function in painful diabetic neuropathy. Journal of the neurological Sciences 74: 1–9

Hollis J B, Castell D O, Braddom R L 1977 Esophageal function in diabetes mellitus and
its relation to peripheral neuropathy. Gastroenterology 73: 1098–1102

Holman R R, White V M, Orde-Pecker C, Steemson J, Smith B, McPherson K, Rizza C,
Knight A H, Dornan T L, Howard-Williams J, Jenkins L, Rolfe R, Barbour D, Poon
P, Mann J I, Bron A J, Turner R C 1983 Prevention of deterioration of renal and
sensory-nerve function by more intensive management of insulin-dependent diabetic
patients: a two-year randomized prospective study. Lancet 1: 204–208

Hosking D J, Moody F, Stewart I M, Atkinson M 1975 Vagal impairment of gastric
secretion in diabetic autonomic neuropathy. British Medical Journal 2: 588–590

Hutchison K J, Johnson B W, Williams H T G, Brown G D 1974 The histamine flare
response in diabetes mellitus. Surgery Gynecology and Obstetrics 139: 566–568

Jakobsen J, Christiansen J S, Kristoffersen I, Christensen C K, Hermnasen K, Schmitz A, Mogensen C E 1988 Autonomic and somatosensory nerve function after 2 years of continuous subcutaneous insulin infusion in Type I diabetes. Diabetes 37: 452–455

Johnson P C, Doll S C, Cromer D W 1986 Pathogenesis of diabetic neuropathy. Annals of Neurology 19: 450–457

Jordan W R 1936 Neuritic manifestations in diabetes mellitus. Archives of Internal Medicine 57: 307–366

Judzewitsch R G, Jaspan J B, Polonsky K S, Weinberg C R, Halter J B, Halar E, Pfeifer M A, Vukadinovic C, Bernstein L, Schneider M, Liang K–Y, Gabbay K H, Rubenstein A H, Porte D 1983 Aldose reductase inhibition improves nerve conduction velocity in diabetic patients. New England Journal of Medicine 308: 119–125

Kennedy W R, Sakuta M, Sutherland D, Goetz F C 1984a Quantitation of the sweating deficiency in diabetes mellitus. Annals of Neurology 15: 482–488

Kennedy W R, Sakuta M, Sutherland D, Goetz F C 1984b The sweating deficiency in diabetes mellitus: methods of quantitation and clinical correlation. Neurology 34: 758–763

Lancet 1989 Diabetic neuropathy 1: 1113–1114

Learmonth J 1953 The surgeon and ischaemia. British Medical Journal 1: 743–748

Le Quesne P M, Fowler C J 1986 A study of pain threshold in diabetics with neuropathic foot lesions. Journal of Neurology, Neurosurgery and Psychiatry 49: 1191–1194

Le Quesne P M, Fowler C J 1987 Quantitative evaluation of toxic neuropathies in man. In: Ellingson R J, Murray N M F, Halliday A M (eds) The London symposium, EEG journal supplement 39: 347–354

Le Quesne P M, Fowler C, Parkhouse N 1990 Peripheral neuropathy profile in various groups of diabetics. Journal of Neurology, Neurosurgery and Psychiatry 53: 558–563

Levy D M, Abraham R R, Abraham R M 1987 Small- and large-fibre involvement in early diabetic neuropathy: a study with the medial plantar response and sensory thresholds. Diabetes Care 10: 441–447

Lewis T 1927 The blood vessels of the human skin and their responses. Shaw and Sons, London

Lewis T 1937 The nocifensor system of nerves and its reactions. Lectures I and II. British Medical Journal 1: 431–435 and 491–494

Lindblom U 1981 Quantitative testing of sensibility including pain. In: Stalberg E, Young R R (eds) Clinical neurophysiology. Butterworths Int Medical Reviews. Butterworth, London, p 168–190

Low P A, Neumann C, Dyck P J, Feeley R D, Tuck R R 1983a Evaluation of skin vasomotor reflexes by using laser Doppler velocimetry. Mayo Clinic Proceedings 58: 583–592

Low P A, Caskey P E, Tuck R R, Fealey R D, Dyck P J 1983b Quantitative sudomotor axon reflex test (Q-SART). Annals of Neurology 14: 573–580

Lynn B, Perl E R 1977 A comparison of four tests for assessing the pain sensitivity of different subjects and test areas. Pain 3: 353–365

Martin M M 1953a Involvement of autonomic nerve fibres in diabetic neuropathy. Lancet 1: 561–565

Martin M M 1953b Diabetic neuropathy. A clinical study of 150 cases. Brain 76: 594–624

Moorhouse J A, Carter S A, Doupe J 1966 Vascular responses in diabetic peripheral neuropathy. British Medical Journal 1: 883–888

Navarro X, Kennedy W R, Fries T J 1989 Small nerve fibre dysfunction in diabetic neuropathy. Muscle and Nerve 12: 498–507

Parkhouse N, Le Quesne P M 1988a Quantitative objective assessment of peripheral nociceptive C fibre function. Journal of Neurology, Neurosurgery and Psychiatry 51: 28–34

Parkhouse N, Le Quesne P M 1988b Impaired neurogenic vascular response in patients with diabetes and neuropathic foot lesions. New England Journal of Medicine 318: 1306–1309

Pirart J 1978 Diabetes mellitus and its degenerative complications, a prospective study of 4400 patients observed between 1947 and 1973. Diabetes Care I: 168–188 and 252–263

Pryce T D 1887 A case of perforating ulcers of both feet with diabetes and ataxic symptoms. Lancet ii: 11–12

Pryce T D 1893 On diabetic neuritis, with a clinical and pathological description of three cases of diabetic pseudotabes. Brain 16: 416–424

Rayman G, Hassan A, Tooke J E 1986 Blood flow in the skin of the foot related to posture in diabetes. British Medical Journal 292: 87–90

Said G, Slama G, Selva J 1983 Progressive centripetal degeneration of axons in small-fibre diabetic neuropathy. A clinical and pathological study. Brain 106: 791–807

Salle H J A, Verberk M M 1984 Comparison of five methods for measurement of vibratory perception. International Archives of Occupational and Environmental Health 53: 303–309

Scarpello J H B, Sladen G E 1978 Progress report: diabetes and the gut. Gut 19: 1153–1162

Service F J, Rizza R A, Daube J R, O'Brien T C, Dyck P J 1985 Near-normoglycaemia improved nerve conduction and vibration sensation in diabetic neuropathy. Diabetologia 28: 722–727

Sidenius P, Jakobsen J 1982 Reversibility and preventability of the decrease in slow axonal transport velocity in experimental diabetes. Diabetes 31: 689–693

Smith S E, Smith S A, Brown P M, Fox C, Sonksen P H 1978 Pupillary signs in diabetic autonomic neuropathy. British Medical Journal 2: 924–927

Sosenko J M, Kato M, Soto R A, Gadia M T, Ayyar D R 1988 Specific assessments of warm and cool sensitivities in adult diabetic patients. Diabetes Care 11: 481–483

Spencer P S, Schaumburg H H 1976 Central-peripheral distal axonopathy — the pathology of dying-back polyneuropathies. Progress in Neuropathology 3: 253–295

Starr I 1930 Studies of the circulation of the feet in diabetes mellitus with and without gangrene. Americal Journal of Medical Science 180: 149–171

Stokes I A, Faris I B, Hutton W C 1975 The neuropathic ulcer and loads on the foot in diabetic patients. Acta Orthopedica Scandinavica 46: 839–47

Sugimura K, Dyck P J 1982 Multifocal fibre loss in proximal sciatic nerve in symmetric distal diabetic neuropathy. Journal of the Neurological Sciences 53: 501–509

Thomas P K 1987 Vascular factors in the causation of diabetic neuropathy. Trends in Neurological Sciences 10: 6–7

Thomas P K, Lascelles R G 1965 Schwann-cell abnormalities in diabetic neuropathy. Lancet i: 1355–1357

Thomas P K, Eliasson S G 1984 Diabetic neuropathy. In: Dyck P J, Thomas P K, Lambert E H, Bunge R (eds) Peripheral neuropathy, 2nd edn, W B Saunders, Philadelphia, p 1773–1810

Thomas P K, Lascelles R G 1966 The pathology of diabetic neuropathy. Quarterly Journal of Medicine 35: 489–509

Timperley W R, Ward J D, Preston F E, Duckworth T, O'Malley B C 1976 Clinical and histological studies in diabetic neuropathy: a reassessment of vascular factors in relation to intravascular coagulation. Diabetologia 12: 237–243

Timperley W R, Boulton A J M, Davies-Jones G A B, Jarratt J A, Ward J D 1985 Small vessel disease in progressive diabetic neuropathy associated with good metabolic control. Journal of Clinical Pathology 38: 1030–1038

Vallbo A B, Hagbarth K E, Torebjork H E, Wallin B G 1979 Somatosensory, proprioceptive, and sympathetic activity in human peripheral nerves. Physiology Reviews 59: 919–957

Vlassara H, Brownlee M, Cerami A 1981 Excessive non-enzymatic glycosylation of peripheral and central nervous system myelin components in diabetic rats. Proceedings of the National Academy of Sciences USA 78: 5190–5192

Ward J D, Boulton A J M, Simms J M, Sandler D A, Knight G 1983 Venous distention in the diabetic neuropathic foot (Physical sign of arteriovenous shunting). Journal of the Royal Society of Medicine 76: 1011–1014

Watkins P J 1973 Facial sweating after food: a new sign of diabetic autonomic neuropathy. British Medical Journal 1: 583–587

Williamson R T 1904 Changes in the spinal cord in diabetes mellitus. British Medical Journal 1: 122–123

Woltman H W, Wilder R M 1929 Diabetes mellitus: pathologic changes in the spinal cord and peripheral nerves. Archives of Internal Medicine 44: 576–603

Wybauw L 1938 Contribution a l'etude du role vasomoteur et trophique des nerfs sensitifs-III, les reflexes axoniques vasodilateurs leur signification functionelles. Archives Internationales de Physiologie et de Biochimie 46: 345–355

Young R J, Zhou Y Q, Rodriquez E, Prescott R J, Ewing D J, Clarke B F 1986 Variable relationship between peripheral somatic and autonomic neuropathy in patients with different syndromes of diabetic polyneuropathy. Diabetes 35: 192–197

Yue D K, Hanwell M A, Satchell P M, Turtle J R 1982 The effect of aldose reductase
inhibition on motor nerve conduction velocity in diabetic rats. Diabetes 31: 789–794
Ziegler D, Mayer P, Gries F A 1988 Evaluation of thermal, pain, and vibration sensation
thresholds in newly diagnosed Type I diabetic patients. Journal of Neurology,
Neurosurgery and Psychiatry 51: 1420–1424

5. Infection and wound healing

The topics infection and wound healing are linked because the ability to mount an inflammatory response is an essential component of both the wound healing process and the mechanisms of resistance to infection. In addition, wound infection is an important cause of failure of wound healing. This chapter discusses the mechanisms that may impair the responses to infection and the process of wound healing in diabetic patients. The bacteriology of the diabetic foot and therapeutic antibiotic regimens will also be discussed.

The increased liability for diabetics to develop infections became part of the conventional wisdom in much the same way as the susceptibility to vascular disease: and as with vascular disease, the beliefs about infection have been challenged. Several large series have demonstrated that diabetes is a risk factor for the development of wound infection following operation (Cruse & Foord 1973). However Howard (1964) concluded that when allowance was made for the age of the subjects the increased risk attributable to diabetes was no longer present. Many diabetics are obese and this, too, predisposes to the development of wound infection. The statistical techniques used in the reported studies have not been adequate to show if diabetes was a primary risk factor independent of, for example, age and obesity. Whatever the true situation, the important practical point is that the risk of infection is not so high as to preclude safe elective surgery on patients with diabetes.

Infection is an important contributing factor to the morbidity of diabetic patients with foot problems, but it is uncertain if they have a greater susceptibility to infection as a result of impaired resistance, or whether reduced blood supply allows infections to become established and the neuropathy permits the infection to go unrecognized. In any case the foot is now the commonest site for infection in diabetics and there is an excess representation of diabetics in groups of patients with deep infections of the foot.

The clinical importance of these infections has been discussed by Gibbons & Eliopoulos (1984) who said: 'It is probable that many of these [major amputations in diabetics] are performed needlessly because of misconceptions about the treatment of foot infections.'

Other forms of infection have been reported to be more common in diabetics. These groups include staphylococcal skin infections (particularly carbuncles), osteomyelitis, non-specific renal infections and renal tuberculosis, and certain fungal infections, e.g. vulval candidiasis. In the pre-antibiotic era, infection was a particularly feared complication of amputation in diabetics and the desire to be free of infected tissue was one of the reasons why high amputations were regularly performed in these patients.

MECHANISMS

The events which begin with an injury and end with the repair of the damage are a continuous sequence in which each successive change is dependent on the satisfactory progress of the preceding changes. However it is convenient to separate the process into discrete sections. Diabetes might lead to the impairment of the inflammatory and wound healing processes by reducing:

1. The blood supply to the affected area
2. The effectiveness of the inflammatory response
3. The repair process which results in the formation of fibrous tissue.

Impairment of blood supply

The pathological changes that occur in blood vessels in diabetes are described in Chapter 3. In atherosclerosis, failure of wound healing is one of the characteristic results of minor injuries. A reduced blood supply may be enough to maintain the viability of tissues protected by an intact skin, but it may not be able to increase sufficiently to permit healing of even small wounds and, as a result, necrosis and infection may follow. The detection of hyperaemia around an ulcer or wound is the basis of one of the special tests used to predict healing of ulcers on the leg and foot (see p. 144). Diabetics who develop severe atherosclerosis are likely to suffer from failure to heal wounds of the leg and foot, in the same way as non-diabetics. In ischaemic tissue the growth of anaerobic organisms is favoured, particularly if there is concomitant growth of aerobes. The risk of gas gangrene following amputation in non-diabetics is well known, but in addition diabetics may develop a spreading myositis produced by non-clostridial anaerobes (see p. 72). This latter infection is only marginally less dangerous than the former.

There are several mechanisms by which changes involving the microcirculation in diabetes could impair the response to injury. Blockage of small blood vessels might prevent the blood flow from increasing sufficiently to allow healing. However, the microvascular disease seen on histological examination is patchy in its distribution and it is considered unlikely that ischaemia due to these changes is a major cause of impaired healing. Denervation of blood vessels might result in a reduced vascular response to injury (see Ch. 4 for details). In addition the response of the denervated vessels to other stimuli may also be abnormal: there is evidence of increased vasoconstriction in response to both catecholamines (denervation hypersensitivity) and cold (see p. 51), and these might provide significant obstacles for the local autoregulatory mechanisms to overcome. These responses may aid the development of infection because there is evidence that local vasoconstriction produced, for example, by injection of adrenaline, enhances the infectivity of bacteria.

Formation of fluid-cellular exudate

The next phase of the inflammatory response is the accumulation at the site of injury of leucocytes to ingest and destroy bacteria, and protein-rich fluid which aids this task. The capillary basement membrane thickening might alter the permeability and thus interfere with leucocyte migration and fluid exudation. These processes can be broken down into a number of stages including transport to the site of inflammation, migration through vessel walls, recognition of the object of phagocytosis, ingestion, killing of bacteria and subsequent digestion of phagocytosed material (Fig. 5.1). The effectiveness of these measures depends not only on the intrinsic activities of the cells but also on complex groups of proteins in the blood which facilitate the processes. There is evidence that several of these stages are impaired in diabetics.

Adherence. Neutrophils adhere preferentially to vascular endothelium adjacent to a site of inflammation. This is due to the presence on the neutrophils of binding sites for the products of the inflammatory response (Johnston 1982). Various morphological and electrophysiological changes in the cells accompany this process which is reduced by corticosteroids.

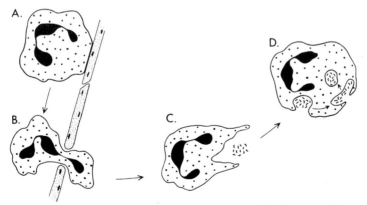

Fig. 5.1 Stages in the cellular response to inflammation. (A.) Adhesion to capillary wall. (B.) Migration through wall. (C.) Progression towards bacteria (Chemotaxis). (D.) Ingestion and destruction of bacteria (Phagocytosis).

Decreased adhesion of polymorphs to vessel walls and reduced rate of escape from vessels have been described in diabetics. It is uncertain whether the defect is in the leucocytes or in the vessel wall. Earlier studies suggested that the level of the blood glucose did not influence these processes. However, using an in vitro system, Bagdade et al (1978) found that the adherence of granulocytes was decreased in hyperglycaemic patients. The abnormality was directly related to the level of fasting blood glucose and returned towards normal with treatment. More recently the same group (Bagdade & Walters 1980) have demonstrated the same effect in patients with milder hyperglycaemia treated with an oral hypoglycaemic agent.

These studies have been extended by the demonstration that the adherence of neutrophils to cultured aortic endothelial cells is reduced (Andersen et al 1988). This group also demonstrated that diabetic serum contained a factor which increased adherence. The interesting implication of these findings is that the cells are abnormal but the serum contains substances that tend to reduce the effect of this abnormality. Alterations in adherence are probably clinically significant because patients with genetic defects of adherence have an increased risk of suffering bacterial infections.

Diapedesis.   This describes the process by which cells squeeze through the junctions between endothelial cells. This process is thought to require glycolysis. Changes in the rheological properties of white cells which may affect diapedesis have been reported in diabetics (Vermes 1987).

Chemotaxis.   Once through the vessel wall the cells move along a chemical gradient. The movement of the cell depends on chemical factors analagous to those in muscle. At a microscopic level, reduced chemotaxis has been associated with a deficiency in the cells of specific granules. It has been suggested that these granules are the source of new membrane and new receptors for characteristic factors which are essential for the movement of the cell.

Chemotaxis is impaired in some diabetics. Mowat & Baum (1971) considered that this change, which was not seen in all subjects, might be genetically determined because it was present in first-degree relatives of patients with diabetes. In addition, abnormalities of chemotaxis could not be demonstrated in cells taken from normal subjects and placed in a hyperglycaemic medium although the defect in the cells could be reversed by incubating with insulin.

Phagocytosis (ingestion) and killing of bacteria   (Fig 5.1). The first step in these processes is the recognition of the foreign material. This is facilitated by the activity of antibodies or other humoral factors, e.g. the complement system. The phagocytic cell then sends out pseudopodia to envelop the organism which comes to lie in a vacuole within the cell. This process is probably a function of receptors on the surface of the cell. The process of killing the bacteria is accompanied by the discharge of enzymes from granules in the cell into the vacuoles containing the bacteria. This is associated with a burst of oxidative activity within the cells which results in the conversion of oxygen to bactericidal products such as superoxide anion, hydrogen peroxide and hydroxyl radical.

The ability of the polymorphs to ingest and kill bacteria is reduced in diabetes (for review see Robertson & Polk 1974). The evidence from several experiments suggests that granulocytes from diabetic patients are normal in their ability to take up bacteria (Dziatkowiak et al 1982). However, these and other authors have demonstrated that the cells are less able to kill ingested bacteria. This defect may be improved but not returned to normal by more rigorous control of the diabetes (Nolan et al 1978). The mechanism of the impairment is almost certainly a reduction in the generation of the bactericidal factors from oxygen. Production of these substances depends on glucose metabolism via the pentose phosphate pathway which is closely connected to the carbohydrate metabolism of the cell. Appropriate metabolic abnormalities can be demonstrated in these cells in diabetic patients.

A very important component of the cellular response is the appearance of mononuclear cells which also have important phagocytic functions. Leibovich & Ross (1975) have demonstrated that impairment of monocyte function seriously impairs fibroblastic activity in experimental animals. Kitahara et al (1980) have shown abnormal metabolic activity in monocytes from diabetics although it is not known if their activity is impaired in vivo.

The effect of ketosis has been studied by several groups with conflicting results. Some have found that ketoacidosis is necessary before abnormalities of leucocyte function can be detected but other workers have demonstrated abnormalities in the absence of ketosis.

The preceding sections have considered the local components of the cellular response to inflammation. Abnormalities have also been demonstrated in several of the systemic components of the response. These include:

1. A smaller increase in neutrophil and monocyte count following exposure to endotoxin (Gilbert et al 1978).

2. A reduction in the number of phagocytosing monocytic cells in diabetics with infection (Katz et al 1983).

3. Impaired function of fixed phagocytic cells of the reticuloendothelial system in diabetics with microvascular disease (Iavicoli et al 1982).

All these changes would tend to increase the susceptibility of diabetic patients to infection.

Formation of fibrous tissue

The changes of the inflammatory response are an essential preliminary to the formation of collagenous fibrous tissue. There is very little clinical evidence that wound healing in the absence of infection is less efficient in diabetics. A number of studies have shown differences between diabetics and non-diabetics in the rate of healing of foot amputations, but in these circumstances the adequacy of the blood supply is of critical importance, and the published series do not always provide the data to assess this point.

The conditions are easier to control in animal experiments. Goodson & Hunt (1979) have reviewed the evidence which suggests that wound healing is impaired in insulin-deficient animals. The earliest changes were examined by Arquilla et al (1976) who found a lack of DNA production close to the wound, reduced new capillary formation and decreased collagen production. These abnormalities were seen within 4 hours of wounding and emphasize the importance of the inflammatory response, abnormalities of which have been described in the previous sections. Insulin deficiency was noted to be associated with fewer granulocytes and fibroblasts, more oedema and fewer capillaries (Weringer et al 1981). They suggested that lack of insulin, rather than hyperglycaemia, was responsible for the impaired capillary growth. The formation of granulation tissue and collagen was studied by Yue et al (1986). They observed that the amount of collagen produced was reduced but the hydroxyproline/proline ratio was normal in diabetic animals. Collagen formation was not enhanced by treatment with an aldose reductase inhibitor. The reduction in granulation tissue was not specific to diabetes but was also found in uraemia and malnutrition. In longer-term studies Goodson & Hunt (1979) and Yue et al (1987) demonstrated that the development of strength in an incised wound, which was closely related to the amount of collagen produced in the tissues closest to the wound edge, was decreased in insulin deficiency. In another animal model, the obese mouse, Goodson and Hunt (1986) demonstrated that poor healing was not restored by insulin administration. They argued that excess adipose tissue was an independent factor in causing poor healing.

It is likely that the effects of insulin deficiency on wound healing are due to the changes which occur in the earliest stages after wounding. The experiments of Goodson & Hunt demonstrated that granulation tissue formation could be returned to normal if insulin was given soon after wounding. If the insulin replacement was delayed until the time of greatest collagen formation (about 10 days after wounding) there was no increase in the amount of collagen formed. This is supported by the observation of Yue et al (1987) that there is a non-linear relationship between glycosylated haemoglobin levels and wound strength, suggesting that near perfect control of the diabetes is necessary. It has been demonstrated in patients (Goodson & Hunt 1984) that insulin treatment restores to normal the accumulation of collagen in a wound. These findings suggest that the greatest care should be taken to control the diabetes in the early postoperative period. In practice this is the time when good control is most difficult to achieve.

Insulin is one of many agents which have been alleged to increase the rate of wound healing when applied topically. However these types of studies face formidable difficulties of design and assessment of outcome. The experimental evidence is against this kind of treatment. Insulin did not increase the healing of granulating wounds in a study by Rosenthal & Enquist (1968) and in tissue culture experiments the rate of collagen synthesis was dependent on the availability of glucose not insulin.

This section has given details of a number of mechanisms by which resistance to infection and wound healing might be impaired and it is probable that both these defects are part of the syndrome of diabetes mellitus. However, the effects of the abnormalities described are largely or totally reversible with treatment and in these circumstances the risks to the patient are not significantly greater than in a non-diabetic subject.

BACTERIOLOGY

The preceding account has discussed the host factors in the resistance to infection. Factors affecting the bacteria may also be important. In vitro, high concentrations of glucose are believed to favour the multiplication of gram-positive bacteria, especially staphylococci, rather than gram-negative organisms. This matches the clinical observation (Robson 1970) that in patients with septicaemia, gram-positive organisms were found in 80% of cases with a blood glucose level of greater than 7.2 mmol/l and gram-negative organisms in a similar proportion of patients with a lower blood glucose. It also supports the clinical observation that staphylococcal skin infections are more common in hyperglycaemic patients so that it is important to test for diabetes mellitus in any patient who presents with a carbuncle or repeated staphylococcal skin infections.

In the foot there are few specific features about the nature of the invading microorganisms. The diabetic may suffer from the same sorts of infections that afflict non-diabetics. The common types include fungus infections of skin or nails. Fungus infections of the skin usually occur in moist areas of the foot and are often associated with poor hygiene. They should be regarded as a warning and an indication for the patient to be reminded of the need for proper care of the feet. The species most commonly involved are *Tricophyton rubrum*, *T. interdigitale* and *Epidermophyton flocculosum*. Paronychia may be due to yeast or staphylococcal infection and may be extensive if the foot is insensitive. Staphylococcal infection will usually require drainage as well as antibiotic therapy.

The deep infections of the foot are the most difficult to manage. In recent years there have been several studies reporting the bacteriological findings in these patients. These have emphasized the need for careful technique in collecting specimens (to avoid contamination from superficial tissues) and the frequency of anaerobic organisms. It is suggested that ulcer curettage or deep-tissue biopsy is the preferred method of obtaining specimens for the culture of the responsible bacteria (McIntyre 1987). The other important observation is that on average there are more than three organisms in each infected foot. The results are summarized in Table 5.1.

Table 5.1 Bacteria cultured from patients with deep infections of the foot

Organism	Frequency %
Aerobic	
Gram-positive	
Staphylococcus aureus	27–46
Staphylococcus epidermidis	32–40
Streptococcus Group A	3–6
Streptococcus Group B	10–20
Streptococcus (other)	6–18
Gram-negative	
Escherischia coli	6–17
Klebsiella pneumoniae	6–10
Proteus mirabilis	10–24
Proteus vulgaris	2–7
Enterobacter spp	8–14
Pseudomonas aeruginosa	7–19
Anaerobic	
Peptostreptococcus spp	7–22
Bacteroides spp	10–26
Clostridia	1–6

Sources: Bamberger et al 1987, Jones et al 1985, Leichter et al 1988, Wheat et al 1986

Rare but lethal infections occur as a result of infection with anaerobic organisms. Spreading anaerobic infection is a serious complication of a wound or foot operation. The detailed clinical features are described on page 158. There are two groups of bacteria involved.

Spore-bearing clostridia

These are the same species, predominantly *Clostridium perfringens*, that cause gas gangrene in non-diabetics (Darke et al 1977). But in more than half the cases additional organisms can be cultured.

Non-clostridial anaerobes

Non-clostridial anaerobic infections can occur in non-diabetics but are more common in diabetics. The organisms responsible, including bacteroides and anaerobic streptococci, are commonly found contaminating lesions on the feet of diabetics. The infection should be differentiated from synergistic gangrene due classically to a combined infection with micro-aerophilic streptococci and *Staphylococcus aureus*. This infection, which characteristically affects the perineum or abdominal wall, causes a spreading skin necrosis.

Therapy of anaerobic infections includes penicillin administration and amputation clear of the infected area. If hyperbaric oxygen therapy is available, it may quickly limit the spread of the infection, the rapidity of the response being characteristic of clostridial infection. If a rapid response is not obtained the infection is unlikely to be clostridial and prolonging the hyperbaric therapy is unlikely to be of benefit (Darke et al 1977). Clostridial infection typically follows a major amputation for ischaemia and is preventable by the preoperative administration of penicillin, which should always be given. For both types of infection it is important to recognize that antibiotic therapy is often insufficient to prevent death and high amputation may be required.

ANTIBIOTIC THERAPY

The major role of antibiotic therapy is to limit the spread of infection (see Table 5.2). This is important in the following circumstances:

1. To prevent the spread of infection around an ulcer or area of gangrene
2. To limit the cellulitis which surrounds an abscess
3. To prevent the establishment of infection following surgery.

Continuing infection will result in progressive loss of tissue and in some cases may make the critical difference between loss of part of the foot, which produces minor disability, and a below-knee amputation, a major disability. The distinction must be made between contamination (or colonization) with bacteria and infection. Bacteria are always present in specimens obtained from open wounds. This is particularly true if there is thick, moist skin around the area of necrotic tissue in the base of the lesion. This does not mean that all patients should be given antibiotics. In most cases antibiotic therapy would be wasted because it is not possible to sterilize an area where dead tissue remains. However, if signs of cellulitis (redness, warmth and swelling) are present antibiotics should not be withheld. It is also important to remember that antibiotic therapy is never sufficient treatment for an abscess; adequate drainage is always required.

Knowledge of the flora in a particular patient is important if appropriate

Table 5.2 Antibiotic therapy of the diabetic foot

Indications
1. Treatment of cellulitis
   a. No abscess: curative
   b. Abscess present: limit spread of infection before drainage
2. Prophylaxis
   a. Before local amputation: broad spectrum
   b. Before major amputation: penicillin

Choice of antibiotics
1. Therapy of infection
   Cefoxitin 1–2 g i.v. 8 hourly
   Metronidazole 200 mg orally or rectally 8 hourly
   Amoxycillin 500 mg orally or i.m. 6 hourly
   Clindamycin 300 mg orally or i.m. 6 hourly
   Lincomycin 600 mg i.m. 6–12 hourly
2. Prophylaxis of gas gangrene
   Penicillin 1 million units (600 mg) i.m. or i.v. 4–6 hourly for 24 hours
   In penicillin-sensitive patients:
      If minor symptoms on prior exposure use cefalothin 1 g i.v.
      If previous major allergic features use erythromycin 300–600 mg i.v. 6 hourly for 24 hours

antibiotic therapy is to be given and specimens should always be taken for culture from patients admitted to hospital for treatment of a foot ulcer even though there may be no immediate indication for antibiotics. The detailed management of a patient with an abscess of the foot is discussed in Chapter 10. An important part of that management is the administration of antibiotics for 24–48 hours before operation. If a serious infection is present antibiotic therapy will be required to combat a wide spectrum of organisms, and in most cases will be given before the results of cultures are available.

The choice of antibiotics for use depends on a knowledge of the types of organisms which may be present and on the clinical severity of the infection. Table 5.2 lists the antibiotics which may be administered and gives their usual doses. If a single agent is to be used, cefoxitin is probably the best because of its activity against bacteroides species as well as the spectrum it shares with the other cephalosporins. Its disadvantage is a relative lack of activity against staphylococci. The combination of amoxycillin with clindamycin or lincomycin may be used: amoxycillin because of its activity against many gram-negative organisms and streptococci (including enterococci), and clindamycin because of its effectiveness against staphylococci and bacteroides. Clindamycin may be given orally and parenteral administration should be used for lincomycin. Penicillin is the agent of choice for the treatment of, or prophylaxis against, clostridial infection. Metronidazole has the advantages of being relatively non-toxic and active after administration either by mouth or by rectum. More recently available antibiotics such as amoxycillin/potassium clavulanate (Augmentin) and quinolones such as cepriofloxacin may prove to be useful in these patients.

Antibiotics are effective at controlling cellulitis. This has two important consequences for the patient. First it minimizes the local tissue damage and second, it reduces the size of the inflammatory focus so that the general condition of the patient improves and the diabetes becomes easier to control.

Prophylactic antibiotics

The principle that antibiotic therapy, given preoperatively, will reduce the incidence of wound infections when the operation is carried out in a contaminated field is well established in surgical practice. Amputation performed close to an ulcer or area of gangrene in a diabetic patient is a very good example of the application of this principle. Freshly opened tissue planes are much more vulnerable to the establishment of infection than areas of granulation tissue. To be of benefit, the antibiotics used must be effective against the likely types of potentially invasive bacteria. The cardinal principle, however, is that the blood must contain an adequate concentration of antibiotics at the time of operation.

Timing is absolutely critical. Antibiotics which, given preoperatively, would reduce the chances of wound infection to low levels are much less effective if their administration is delayed for as little as 4 hours. This means that while antibiotics given 1 hour before the operation are likely to be effective, it is often too late to give the same agents when the patient is in the recovery room after surgery.

The other important practical point which has followed from observations is that the duration of antibiotic therapy, when used prophylactically, may be shorter than when established infection is being treated: 12–24 hours for prophylaxis compared with a 5 day course for treatment of infection. However the conditions in the wound following, for example, a ray amputation (see p. 165) in a diabetic patient are different from those following, say, elective colectomy for neoplasm of the colon. In the latter case there may have been a heavy contamination dose of bacteria during the operation, but this risk is decreased when the anastomosis is completed and the skin wound closed. In the open wound on the diabetic foot, however, bacteria may multiply on the dressings while the exposed tissues are vulnerable to infection before granulation tissue forms. Because the foot is vulnerable for a longer time the course of antibiotics is often continued for 5 days. The use of antibiotics in prophylaxis of gas gangrene has been mentioned above.

REFERENCES

Andersen B, Goldsmith G H, Spagnuolo P J 1988 Neutrophil adhesive dysfunction in diabetes mellitus: the role of cellular and plasma factors. Journal of Laboratory and Clinical Medicine 111: 275–285

Arquilla E R, Weringer E J, Nakajo M 1976 Wound healing: a model for the study of diabetic angiopathy. Diabetes 25: 811–819

Bagdade J D, Stewart M, Walters E 1978 Impaired granulocyte adherence: a reversible defect in host defence in patients with poorly controlled diabetes. Diabetes 27: 677–681

Bagdade J D, Walters E 1980 Impaired granulocyte adherence in mildly diabetic patients: effects of tolazamide treatment. Diabetes 29: 309–311

Bamberger D M, Daus G P, Gerding D N 1987 Osteomyelitis in the feet of diabetic patients. American Journal of Medicine 83: 653–660

Cruse P J E, Foord R 1973 A five-year prospective study of 23 649 surgical wounds. Archives of Surgery 107: 206–210

Darke S G, King A M, Slack W K 1977 Gas gangrene and related infections: classification, clinical features and aetiology, management and mortality. A report of 88 cases. British Journal of Surgery 64: 104–112

Dziatkowiak H, Kowalska M, Denys A 1982 Phagocytic and bactericidal activity of granulocytes in diabetic children. Diabetes 31: 1041–1043

Gibbons G W, Eliopoulos G M 1984 Infection of the diabetic foot. In Kozak G P et al (eds) Management of diabetic foot problems. W B Saunders, Philadelphia, p 97–102

Gilbert H S, Rayfield E J, Smith H, Keusch G T 1978 Effects of acute endotoxaemia and glucose administration on circulating lymphocyte populations is normal in diabetic subjects. Metabolism 27: 889–899

Goodson W H, Hunt T K 1979 Wound healing and the diabetic patient. Surgery, Gynecology and Obstetrics 149: 600–608

Goodson W H, Hunt T K 1984 Wound healing in well-controlled diabetic men. Surgical Forum 35: 614–616

Goodson W H, Hunt T K 1986 Wound collagen accumulates in obese hyperglycaemic mice. Diabetes 35: 491–495

Howard J M 1964 Ad Hoc Committee. Postoperative wound infections: the influence of ultraviolet irradiation of the operating room and various other factors. Annals of Surgery 160 (Suppl)

Iavicoli M, DiMario U, Pozzilli P, Canalese J, Ventriglia L, Galfo C, Andreani D 1982 Impaired phagocytic function and increased immune complexes in diabetics with severe microangiopathy. Diabetes 31: 7–11

Johnston R B 1982 Disorders of neutrophil function. New England Journal of Medicine 307: 434–436

Jones E W, Edwards R, Finch R, Jeffcoate W J 1985 A microbiological study of diabetic foot lesions. Diabetic Medicine 2/3: 213–215

Katz S, Klein B, Elian I, Fishman P, Djaldetti M 1983 Phagocytic activity of monocytes from diabetic patients. Diabetes Care 6: 479–482

Kitahara M, Eyre H J, Lynch R E, Rallison M L, Hill H R 1980 Metabolic activity of diabetic monocytes. Diabetes 29: 251–256

Leibovich S J, Ross R 1975 The role of the macrophage in wound repair. A study with hydrocortisone and antimacrophage serum. American Journal of Pathology 78: 71–100

Leichter S B, Allweiss P, Harley J, Clay J, Kuperstein-Chase J, Sweeney G J, Kolkin J 1988 Clinical characteristics of diabetic patients with serious pedal infections, Metabolism 37 (suppl 1): 22–24

McIntyre K E 1987 Control of infection in the diabetic foot: the role of microbiology, immunopathology, antibiotics and guillotine amputation. Journal of Vascular Surgery 5: 787–790.

Mowat A G, Baum J 1971 Chemotaxis of polymorphonuclear leukocytes from patients with diabetes mellitus. New England Journal of Medicine 284: 621–627

Nolan C M, Beaty H M, Bagdade J D 1978 Further characterization of the impaired bactericidal function of granulocytes in patients with poorly controlled diabetes. Diabetes 27: 889–894

Robertson H D, Polk H C 1974 The mechanism of infection in patients with diabetes mellitus: a review of leukocyte malfunction. Surgery 75: 123–128

Robson M C 1970 A new look at diabetes mellitus and infection. American Journal of Surgery 120: 681–682

Rosenthal D P, Enquist I F 1968 The effect of insulin on granulating wounds in normal animals. Surgery 64: 1096–1098

Vermes I 1987 Rheological properties of white cells are changed in diabetic patients with microvascular complications. Diabetelogia 30: 434–6

Weringer E J, Kelso J M, Tamai I Y, Arquilla E R 1981 The effect of antisera to insulin, 2-deoxyglucose-induced hyperglycaemia and starvation on wound healing in normal mice. Diabetes 30: 407–410

Wheat L J, Allen S D, Henry M, Kernek C B, Siders J A, Kuebler T, Fineberg N, Norton J 1986 Diabetic foot infections: Bacteriologic analysis. Archives of Internal Medicine 146: 1935–1940

Yue D K, Swanson B, McLennan S, Marsh M, Spaliviero J, Delbridge L, Reeve T, Turtle J R 1986 Abnormalities of granulation tissue and collagen formation in experimental diabetes, uraemia and malnutrition. Diabetic Medicine 3: 221–225

Yue D K, McLennan S, Marsh M, My Y W, Spaliviero J, Delbridge L, Reeve T, Turtle J R 1987 Effects of experimental diabetes, anaemia and malnutrition on wound healing. Diabetes 36: 295–299

6. Mechanical factors

The important role of physical factors in the development of ulcers has been mentioned in Chapter 2. The agents involved are largely mechanical although thermal and chemical factors may occasionally be important. The effect of all these agents is aided by and may depend on loss of perception of pain in the foot. Mechanical forces (Fig. 6.1) may act by:

1. Disrupting tissue
2. Pressure causing ischaemia
3. Repetitive stress causing necrosis.

Disruption

Localized high pressure may cause disruption of tissue. A large force is required and this must be applied to a small area. Treading on broken glass or a drawing pin are examples of this sort of force. The best way that a patient can protect himself is always to wear footwear, so that the chance of these accidents is much reduced.

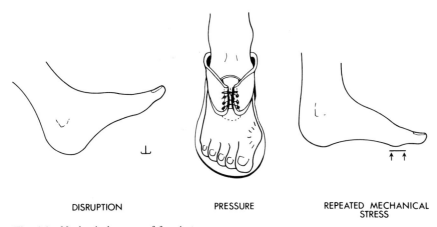

DISRUPTION   PRESSURE   REPEATED MECHANICAL STRESS

Fig. 6.1 Mechanical causes of foot lesions.

Ischaemic necrosis from pressure

On standing, the pressure between some parts of the foot and the surface will be sufficient to stop the blood supply to those areas. Another example of this phenomenon is seen in contracting muscle, e.g. the heart, when the tension developed during contraction stops perfusion. This is normal and harmless. However, if moderate pressure is applied to an area of skin for a prolonged period, ischaemic necrosis of this area may result. One common example is the formation of a bedsore.

This is an important mechanism for the development of lesions in diabetic patients. The forces required are not high, 7–14 kPa is sufficient (Brand 1978), but must be maintained for several hours. If the arterial supply is reduced the pressure required to stop the skin circulation will be less thus atherosclerosis is an additional predisposing factor. There are two situations in which ischaemic necrosis commonly occurs in diabetics. The first is trauma from wearing a new pair of shoes (see Fig. 6.2). The lesions occur on the forefoot, involving the toes and/or bony prominences such as the first metatarsal head, the interphalangeal joint of the great toe and the base of the fifth metatarsal bone. Because the duration of the pressure is critical in the production of necrosis, adequate preventative measures are obvious and simple: new shoes should never be worn for longer than 2 hours until they are well adjusted to the shape of the foot. At the end of this time the shoes and socks should be removed and the feet carefully inspected. Affected areas will be pale initially but the skin reddens as reactive hyperaemia develops. The appearance of such an area means that the particular pair of shoes should not be worn again that day. The second situation in which

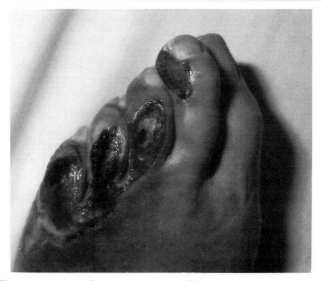

Fig. 6.2 The consequences of wearing new shoes all day.

ischaemic necrosis occurs is in a patient with decreased sensation in the feet who is in bed for a prolonged period. The feet are suffering prolonged application of low pressure. Lesions occur predominantly on the pressure areas around the heel and malleoli. The presence of occlusive arterial disease also potentiates the development of ischaemic necrosis in these patients. Prevention depends on diligent nursing which gives regular attention to pressure areas.

Repetitive stress

The idea that lesions might be produced by moderate repetitive stress, with pressures which neither disrupt the tissues nor cause ischaemic necrosis, has made much clearer our understanding of the development of the common neuropathic ulcer (Brand 1978, Delbridge et al 1985). This concept provides a coherent explanation for the sequence of events leading to the development of an ulcer. A detailed account of the factors involved is given because of its importance and because a unified account of the various factors cannot easily be found elsewhere. The following account is in two parts:

1. The mechanics of walking
2. Abnormalities in diabetes that lead to the formation of ulcers.

MECHANICS OF THE FOOT

When man assumed the erect posture the foot became subject to a variety of stresses which were not encountered by his arboreal ancestors. The evolutionary and adaptive processes are neither complete nor perfect, e.g. the lateral metatarsal bones may fracture with repeated minor trauma (stress fractures). Analysis of the functions of the lower limb during walking has proved difficult although a large number of techniques have been brought to bear including gross anatomical studies, electromyography, cineradiology, cinematography and engineering approaches to the study of load. It is the purpose of this section to consider the mechanical forces on the foot, the abnormalities that may occur in diabetics and the way which the stresses may be modified in the treatment of these patients.

The movements of the ankle and associated joints will only be mentioned briefly and more proximal joints not discussed at all in this account.

Anatomical factors

A casual glance at skin of the foot will immediately reveal one of the most important adaptations for weight bearing, namely the production of keratin. The keratin is thickest on those parts of the foot that carry the greatest load and this is especially noticeable on the heel. Keratin production adapts very quickly to changed loads: it will increase during a seaside holiday if one walks barefoot and will decrease if the leg is immobilized in plaster, with the result that on resumption of walking the skin is soft and tender. If an area of abnormal load develops, e.g. as a result of neuropathic change in an underlying joint, the response is for excess keratin to develop at that site. This is a normal response to increased load.

The subcutaneous tissue is dense with many fibrous bands between the lobules of fat. It is also very strong and resistant to acute trauma, e.g. a fall may result in a fracture of the calcaneum but the overlying skin appears undamaged. However, repeated abnormal stress may result in atrophy of the subcutaneous tissue so that the underlying bones come to lie closer to the skin.

The bones, ligaments and fasciae of the foot are of fundamental importance in walking and their functional anatomy has been studied by many people. The longitudinal arches formed by the tarsal and metatarsal bones differ in several important ways from architectural arches. First, the arches of the foot are flexible and change their shape when under load. Second, the stresses on the arches of the foot produce bending stresses on the plantar aspect whereas on a masonry arch there are purely compressive forces acting. This fact is easily confirmed anatomically by the relative thickness of the plantar as compared to the dorsal ligaments of the foot. The plantar aponeurosis has an important role in preventing excessive displacement of the pillars of the arches — the calcaneum and the metatarsal heads. Much attention has been given to the so-called windlass action of this fascia (see Fig. 6.3). The anterior attachments of the fascia are in the digits so that when the toes are dorsiflexed, as they are during walking just before the foot leaves the ground, there is increased tension in the fascia and this tends to bring closer the pillars of the arch. Fixed shortening of this fascia which may occur in diabetics as a result of dorsal displacement of the toes (see p. 119) may result in a permanently high-arched foot (pes cavus). This has the additional effect of increasing the loads carried by the area of the metatarsal heads. Studies of the load carried by the foot produce no

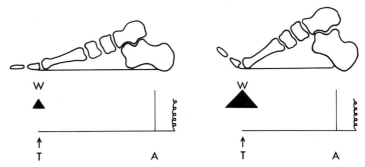

Fig. 6.3 Figure showing (above) how fixed dorsiflexion of the toes results in shortening of the longitudinal arch through the attachments of the plantar fascia. (Below) If the distance TA is shortened a given force applied to the spring will result in a greater load at T.

evidence for the idea of a functionally important transverse arch at the level of the metatarsal heads — indeed it is often true that the middle metatarsals carry greater loads than the first and fifth bones. The actions of the muscles inserting in the foot may be different during walking to those inferred from a study of their attachments in the cadaver. An account of some of these actions is given in the following section.

Gait

The investigation of the mechanics of walking includes two groups of observations. These are the study of the geometry of the changes which occur in the leg and foot and the analysis of the forces exerted. Walking involves the coordinated action of many parts of the body, particularly of the lower limbs. This account is confined to a description of the action directly affecting the foot.

A walking cycle is defined as the time between the heel making contact with the ground and the time immediately before the same heel again makes contact with the ground. Each foot is in contact with the ground for about 60% of the walking cycle. Thus both feet are in contact with the ground from 0–10% of the cycle and from 50–60% of the cycle. The time during which the foot is in contact with the ground can be divided into three parts (Fig. 6.4).

1. *Heel strike.* This begins when the heel strikes the ground and ends when the forefoot comes into contact with the surface.

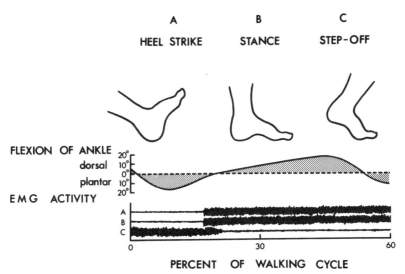

Fig. 6.4 The three phases of gait which occur while the foot is in contact with the ground. The lowest tracings illustrate the electrical activity in: (A.) posterior calf muscles (B.) intrinsic muscles of the foot (C.) anterior calf muscles.

2. *Stance*. This is the longest of the periods and lasts while both heel and forefoot are in contact with the surface. It includes the time when the body weight is transferred forwards and ends when the heel leaves the ground.

3 *Step-off*. During this last phase the body weight is propelled forwards. The forefoot carries its greatest loads during this phase which ends when the foot leaves the ground.

The major movements of the ankle joint and foot are initiated by muscles which arise in the calf. Figure 6.4 shows a simplified version of the events during walking. The position of the ankle joint and the electrical activity of the major muscle groups are shown. During the heel-strike phase there is a plantar flexion of the ankle joint which returns to a neutral position when the forefoot reaches the ground. These movements of the ankle are under the influence of gravity and the anterior tibial muscles. While the foot is in contact with the ground there is progressive dorsiflexion of the ankle as the body weight is transferred forwards. This process is initiated by the anterior tibial muscles, continued by gravity and resisted by the posterior tibial and intrinsic foot muscles. During the step-off phase there is progressive plantar flexion of the ankle until the foot is lifted from the ground.

Denervation of the tibial muscles is seldom a problem in diabetics although, in severe cases of neuropathy, foot drop may occur due to lesions of the common peroneal nerve. More often the gait is ataxic because of sensory neuropathy which affects the joint position sense, so that the precision with which the movements are performed is less. The intrinsic muscles of the foot, although not of great strength, have very important functions in modulating the action of the long flexor and extensor muscles. The extensor digitorum brevis and flexor digitorum accessorius muscles respectively, influence the direction of action of the extensor digitorum longus and flexor digitorum longus muscles. As in the hand, the lumbrical and interosseous muscles cause flexion of the metatarsophalangeal joint and extension of the interphalangeal joint.

The intrinsic muscles have other functions which aid the maintenance of the integrity of the foot. They provide bulk and padding to cover the bones; they help maintain the arches; they provide the maximum surface area for the forefoot; and they limit overextension of the metatarsophalangeal joints.

FORCES UNDER THE FOOT

The forces between the foot and the shoe or ground with which it is in contact comprise both perpendicular or weight-bearing forces and horizontal or frictional forces. Much more is known about the weight-bearing forces because they are much easier to measure than the frictional forces. The studies of weight-bearing described below have helped to explain the distribution and occurrence of plantar ulceration.

The loads carried on the under-surface of the foot depend on body weight and the anatomical and functional properties of the foot, such as the action of the muscles and the bony skeleton (and any abnormalities thereof). The loads are difficult to study precisely. Two types of methods have been used to obtain quantitative data. In the first a load-sensitive area is set into a walkway, so that the forces exerted can be recorded during a single step or while standing. The objection to this method is that the loads recorded might not accurately reflect the forces acting between the foot and any footwear normally worn. This objection is overcome by placing transducers beneath the foot, inside the footwear. However this method has the limitations that only selected areas can be studied and, more important, the presence of transducers might affect the loads measured. Despite these limitations important information has been obtained using both techniques.

For a semi-quantitative study of relative loads the Harris mat has been used. This comprises a rubber mat with ridges at three different levels. The mat is inked and covered with paper on which the subject walks. The arrangement of the ridges is such that the densest impression is produced by the greatest load. This can be used either on the floor or a thin piece of the material can be placed inside the shoe. The latter method gives an idea of the load carried during walking in the patient's own shoe and is likely to be a good guide to the stresses which the foot undergoes during daily activities. This technique has the great advantages of simplicity and ease of interpretation.

The most detailed information has been obtained from studies using a force plate. The measuring system has evolved from a series of parallel beams which enabled the load to be studied on 'slices' of the foot (Stokes et al 1974), through a matrix of 128 cells in an area measuring 12.5 × 25 cm (Hutton & Dhandendran 1979, Fig. 6.5), to the most modern systems in which the loads on the whole area can be estimated (Betts et al 1980). These methods have allowed the study of the dynamic forces during the walking cycle.

When considering the loads carried, the foot may be arbitrarily divided into three areas: heel, midfoot and forefoot. In Figure 6.5 the forefoot has been further subdivided into separate areas for the distal part of the metatarsals and the toes.

Heel.   The load on the heel rises rapidly to high levels (300–400 N) but falls to zero as the load is transferred to the forefoot.

Midfoot.   The midfoot includes the highest parts of the longitudinal arches. In a study of normal subjects the load carried by the midfoot was never greater than 10% of the body weight (Stokes at al 1974). This contradicts the conventional accounts which describe the transfer of the load as occurring along the lateral side of the foot.

Forefoot.   The toes normally carry about 30% of the body weight

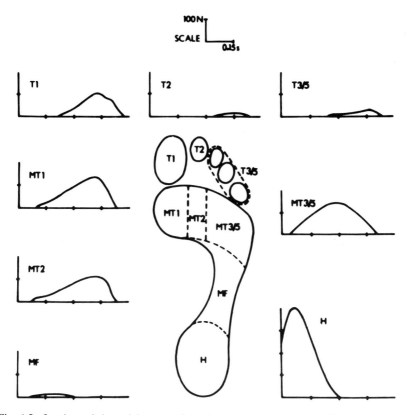

Fig. 6.5 Loads carried on eight areas of the foot during a single step. (Hutton & Dhandendran 1979)

during the later stages of the step-off phase. In normal subjects measurement of the maximum force has shown that the area of the 3rd–4th metatarsal heads carries a load equivalent to 35% of body weight. The great toe and first and second metatarsal separately, carry a maximum of 25% of body weight. The second and third to fifth toes carry less than 10% of body weight.

Similar findings have been reported by Bauman et al (1963) who attached transducers to five sites on the sole of the foot. These transducers were only 1 mm thick so that the distortion produced would be minimal. Their important contribution was to compare barefoot walking on different surfaces with walking using various types of footwear. They demonstrated that the loads measured from a particular area of the foot were less if the subject trod on leather than if the surface was concrete and least when on a rubber surface. Part of this difference might have been artefact due to the varying response of the transducer but there probably remained a real difference between the surfaces. They were also able to demonstrate differences in load carried by the areas of the foot when footwear of different patterns was worn. These findings will be discussed in more detail when the design of shoes is being considered (p. 103).

Frictional forces have been studied by Pollard et al (1983) who attached thin transducers to the sole of the foot to measure horizontal and longitudinal shearing forces. In normal subjects they demonstrated a forward force under the heel and both longitudinal and transverse forces under the metatarsal heads. These forces occurred at areas of maximum vertical load. They also studied the forces with different types of footwear. A plaster cast (see p. 108) minimized the vertical, longitudinal and horizontal forces which were also significantly reduced by Plastazote insoles (see p. 104). A rocker shoe (Fig 7.7) produced a small reduction in vertical load and a larger reduction in longitudinal (but not transverse) shearing forces under the metatarsal heads.

The distribution of body weight when standing has been the subject of conflicting accounts. Hutton et al (1976) demonstrated that there was a range of patterns which might be adopted, all compatible with comfortable stance. The heel carried between one and three times the load carried on the forefoot, but the distribution of the load varied with the need to maintain balance.

CHANGES IN DIABETICS

The alterations which occur in diabetics in the loading of the foot are primarily the result of neuropathy, although partial amputation of the foot may also produce effects equally as important. The effects of neuropathy have been discussed in detail in Chapter 4. The important results are deformities produced by paralysis of the small muscles of the foot and by neuropathic degeneration of the joints. The former produces the claw-toe deformity and the latter may produce areas of high load in abnormal sites. They may have the important results of changing the distribution of forces under the foot. An understanding of these changes would not only help to explain the occurrence and distribution of foot ulcers, but also might direct attention to the sites which are at greatest risk for the development of ulcers.

There are several important conclusions to be drawn from the study of loading on the foot in diabetics.

1. The site of the ulcer always corresponds to the area of the forefoot that carries the highest load (Stokes et al 1975, Ctercteko et al 1981, Boulton et al 1983). In patients whose feet have been deformed either by the presence of neuropathic joints or as a result of operation, e.g. ray amputation, abnormally high loads can be demonstrated over either the deformity (Fig. 6.6) or one or more prominent metatarsal heads (Stokes et al 1975, Fig. 6.7) In feet without ulcers, areas of abnormally high load can be demonstrated, corresponding to the site of callus formation.

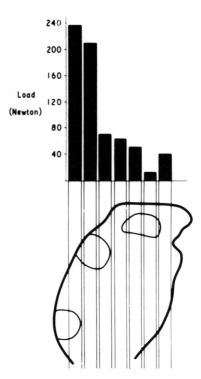

Fig. 6.6 Abnormal loading pattern in a right foot which was deformed by neuropathic degeneration in the tarsal bones. There were ulcers present in both the areas represented by circles on the medial side of the foot.

Examination to seek these areas of high load may be an important part of the surveillance of these patients and modification of the loading pattern might prevent the formation of ulcers. Unfortunately the measuring equipment is expensive and is not widely available.

2. The maximum load is directly proportional to the body weight so that heavier patients may run greater risks of developing foot ulcers.

3. There is a reduction in the load carried by the toes (Ctercteko et al 1981) so that the metatarsal heads carry greater loads. This also means that the toes have lost their main function so that amputation can be performed, if necessary, without further impairment of the function of the foot.

4. Maximum longitudinal shearing forces occur at the sites of healed ulcers (Pollard et al 1983).

Changes in connective tissue

The process of non-enzymic glycosylation by which glucose molecules

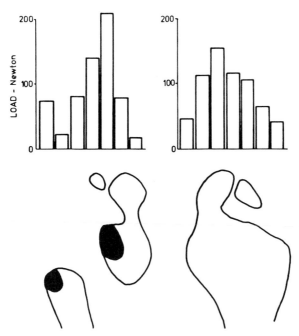

Fig. 6.7   Abnormal loading pattern in a patient following two ray amputations. Both the shaded areas which carried high loads subsequently became ulcers. The pattern for the right foot was normal.

attach to a variety of proteins is now known to be widespread in diabetics. It was first observed with haemoglobin and the estimation of glycosylated haemoglobin is now used as an important indicator of the control of the diabetes (see p. 91). These chemical changes may result in alterations in the physical properties of the protein. A concise account of the processes as they may affect the foot has been given by Delbridge et al (1985) and is summarized below. Glycosylation of collagen makes the tissue less flexible and resistant to digestion by collagenase (Hamlin et al 1975). Together with glycosylation of keratin these changes may produce thickening of the skin and limitation of the mobility of the joints (see p. 98).

Glycosylation of structural proteins in the skin and subcutaneous tissue may contribute to the development of neuropathic ulcers in the following ways:

1. Glycosylated keratin may be resistant to removal and may contribute to the build up of keratin which precedes and accompanies ulceration (see below).

2. The inflexibility of the collagen may potentiate tissue breakdown in areas exposed to high shearing forces (see p. 85). This may facilitate the formation of cavities and eventually ulcers.

The development of neuropathic ulcers

The sequence of events that leads to foot ulcers in diabetics can be reconstructed. One or more areas of the forefoot, in the region of the metatarsal heads or the interphalangeal joint of the great toe, come to carry greater than normal loads. This increase occurs for several reasons:

1. The clawing of the toes means that they are unable to carry their normal load and thus the effective weight-bearing surface of the forefoot is reduced in area.

2. Paralysis and atrophy of the small muscles of the foot results in increased prominence of the metatarsal heads.

3. The lever effect due to shortening of the foot may be important in some cases. The pes cavus deformity is sometimes seen and this change in leverage may be important in these patients (Fig. 6.2). However, more frequently there is no obvious pes cavus presumably because the plantar fascia also gives way under the stress of the loads carried. The clawing also makes the toes more vulnerable to frictional forces.

4. Ctercteko (1982) has suggested that a further factor is the high prevalence of skeletal abnormalities in these patients. These may arise congenitally or from previous injury or surgery.

The link between increased load and the development of ulcers has been given by Brand (1978) who demonstrated that moderate stress applied repeatedly to hand or foot caused inflammation. The force needed was not large and those measured by Stokes et al (1975) were in the range which would produce these effects. In human subjects, Brand demonstrated that these stresses caused redness and tenderness which took more than 24 hours to resolve so that there was reduced tolerance of similar stresses the next day. Daily exposure to these forces in experimental animals produced continued inflammation and eventually necrosis and ulceration of the affected area.

A similar sequence is very likely in the feet of diabetics who, for reasons given above, develop areas of local increase in the load carried. A foot which has normal sensation and which experiences these stresses is protected because the inflammation causes pain. As a result, the subject relieves the stress either by resting or by altering the gait to reduce the load on the tender area. If the patient is unaware of this inflammation because of diabetic or other neuropathy, no action will be taken to relieve the load so that the stresses produced by walking continue, and the progression to necrosis and ulceration may occur. It is difficult to detect these areas in patients, but detection is an important contribution to the prevention of ulceration because, if adequate rest is given, resolution can occur. These areas can be seen as 'hot spots' on thermograms of the foot and their course followed by this method. Skin temperature increases of around 2°C are found in these patients and can be detected by palpation. It must be remembered that many patients have impairment of sensation in their hands as well as their feet. In these cases the feet should be palpated by another person who (presumably) has normal sensation. If more precision is required a thermistor is a sufficiently accurate method for measuring skin temperature.

Details of the subsequent events have been given by Delbridge et al (1985). In response to the stresses described, a plaque of keratin develops and beneath this tissue breakdown occurs as described above. Both these changes may be potentiated by glycosylation of connective tissue proteins in the skin. The cavity which forms enlarges gradually and finally discharges through the skin (Fig. 6.8). The sign of imminent discharge is blood staining of the callus. Once ulceration has occurred there is bacterial contamination and invasive infection may result. Regularly removing the excess keratin (p. 101) is an important step in the prevention and treatment of ulcers.

This chapter has emphasized the importance of mechanical factors as the cause of ulcers in patients with the predisposing factors of ischaemia and/or neuropathy. The next chapter outlines steps to minimize the effects of these causative mechanisms.

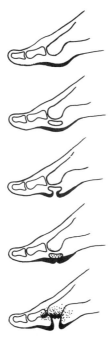

Fig. 6.8 Stages in the development of neuropathic ulceration. (Delbridge et al 1985 by permission of Butterworth & Co).

REFERENCES

Bauman J H, Girling J P, Brand P W 1963 Plantar pressures and trophic ulceration. Journal of Bone and Joint Surgery 45B: 652–673

Betts R P, Franks C I, Duckworth T, Burke J 1980 Static and dynamic foot pressure measurements in clinical orthopaedics. Medical and Biological Engineering and Computing 18: 674–684

Boulton A J M, Hardisty C A, Betts R C, Franks C I, Worth R C, Ward J D, Duckworth T 1983 Dynamic foot pressure and other studies as diagnostic and management aids in diabetic neuropathy. Diabetes Care 6: 26–33

Brand P W 1978 Pathomechanics of diabetic (neutrophic) ulcer and its conservative management. In: Bergan J J and Yao J S T (eds) Gangrene and severe ischaemia of the lower extremities. Grune and Stratton, New York

Ctercteko G 1982 Neuropathic lesions of the diabetic foot. MD Thesis, Sydney University

Ctercteko G C, Dhanendran M, Hutton W C, LeQuesne L P 1981 Vertical forces acting on the feet of diabetic patients with neuropathic ulceration. British Journal of Surgery 68: 608–614

Delbridge L, Ctercteko G, Fowler C, Reeve T S, LeQuesne L P 1985 The aetiology of diabetic neuropathic ulceration of the foot. British Journal of Surgery 72: 1–6

Hamlin C R, Kohn R R, Luschin J H 1975 Apparent accelerated ageing of human collagen in diabetes mellitus. Diabetes 24: 902–904

Hutton W C, Stott J R R, Stokes I A F 1976 The mechanics of the foot. In: Klenerman L (ed) The foot and its disorders. Blackwell, Oxford, p 30–48

Hutton W C, Dhandendran M 1979 A study of the distribution of load under the normal foot during walking. International Orthopaedics 3: 153–157

Pollard J P, LeQuesne L P, Tappin J W 1983 Forces under the foot. Journal of Biomedical Engineering 5: 37–40

Stokes I A F, Stott J R R, Hutton W C 1974 Force distributions under the foot — a dynamic measuring system. Biomedical Engineering 9: 140–143

Stokes I A F, Faris I, Hutton W C 1975 The neuropathic ulcer and loads on the foot in diabetic patients. Acta orthopaedica Scandinavica 46: 839–847

7. Prevention of major lesions

It is a major aim of the management of diabetics to prevent the development of complications of the disease including foot lesions. This aim too frequently fails and later chapters of the book will be concerned with the assessment and management of these failures. This chapter will consider the measures which may be taken to minimize the chances of development of a major lesion. The measures to be discussed include:

1. Routine care given to all diabetic patients
2. Details of the treatment of minor lesions and the non-operative treatment of ulcers
3. Provision of adequate footwear and the use of orthoses.

An account of the ways in which mechanical forces may affect the foot has been given in the preceding chapter and the avoidance of these injuries is the prime topic of this section. This is, however, an appropriate time to consider the vexed question of the effect of control of the blood glucose concentration on the development of complications. Some of the arguments have been discussed in the chapters describing the individual complications of diabetes but a summary of the evidence is presented here.

ROUTINE CARE

Control of the diabetes

There is unanimous agreement that diabetes should be carefully controlled. However two major problems are encountered immediately. The first is to define and assess good control and the second is to demonstrate a resulting benefit. Perfect control of diabetes would be defined as maintaining the blood sugar at the same level as in a healthy non-diabetic. This aim will not be achievable until insulin delivery systems are available that respond to blood glucose levels. It is a matter of opinion as to how much deviation from the ideal state is allowable. Good control may be defined by setting acceptable levels of the blood glucose before and after meals but it must be remembered that blood sugar measurements taken at infrequent intervals do not indicate previous or subsequent fluctuations in concentration.

Great interest has been shown in the observation that glucose may become attached to the haemoglobin molecule to form a separately identifiable substance called haemoglobin AIC (see p. 34). The process involves condensation of the glucose molecule with the N-terminal amino acids of the beta chain of the haemoglobin molecule. The rate of the reaction is a function of the blood glucose concentration. It occurs slowly (and is therefore reversed slowly) and continues for the life of the red cell. Thus the concentration of glycosylated haemoglobin in the blood might give some indication of the mean level of blood glucose over a period of weeks or months, related to the life of the red blood cell (see Koenig & Cerami 1980 for review). In contrast a single estimate of the blood glucose level provides only a brief glimpse of a rapidly changing scene. The estimation of glycosylated haemoglobin provides evidence about the control of diabetes which cannot be obtained from other sources, short of continuous monitoring of blood glucose (Nathan et al 1984). However it should be remembered that there are wide differences between individuals in the rate of formation of glycosylated haemoglobin and in the response to the restoration of normoglycaemia (Brooks et al 1980). Traditional estimates of control, based on blood glucose determinations and clinical assessment, vary considerably from estimates based on measurement of glycosylated haemoglobin. The method is particularly valuable in the management of the young diabetic (Goldstein 1984). It is theoretically possible to maintain glycosylated haemoglobin levels within the normal range, but in practice the average level obtained is still above the normal range despite intensive therapy.

Control and complications

The issue of the greatest importance to diabetic patients is whether perfect control of hyperglycaemia will prevent the development of complications. Despite many years of effort it is still not possible to give a definite answer to this question. An early review was published by Tchobroutsky (1978) and the current state of knowledge summarized by Skyler (1989). There is now good evidence that meticulous control of glycaemia can result in improvement in nerve conduction and slowing of the rate of progression of renal disease. However, there is some worrying evidence that glycaemic control must be achieved early in the disease if retinopathy is to be prevented. Further, in Chapter 3 it was pointed out that there are many factors involved in the development of both atherosclerosis and microvascular disease, and hyperglycaemia is only one of these.

The difficulty of this problem can be seen by the controversy that followed the publication of a policy statement by the American Diabetic Association which concluded: 'the weight of the evidence, particularly that accumulated in the past five years, strongly supports the concept that the microvascular complications of diabetes are decreased by reduction of blood glucose concentration', (Cahill et al 1976). This produced a vigorous response (Siperstein et al 1977) which concluded that 'we have yet to find clear evidence that insulin therapy, as currently applied, has altered the course of the microangiopathic lesions of diabetes'. Skyler (1989) has summarized the issues concisely:

1. There is a relationship between control of hyperglycaemia and complications.
2. Improved control may lessen complications.
3. The degree of control and the time at which control must be instituted so as to lower complications is not known.
4. It is not known if any available method can achieve the level or control which may be needed.

Attempts to produce perfect control of diabetes are not without risks. Hypoglycaemia is the most serious of these. It is the most frequent complication of longstanding diabetes and may have disastrous socioeconomic effects affecting, for example, employment and the obtaining of a driving licence. It may cause short and long-term neurological damage. When insulin pumps are used there is an increased risk of keto-acidosis. This may occur despite continued function of the pump. There will also be additional costs to the patient and/or the community from the extra medical care needed to supervize the control of diabetes. However, in the face of the huge financial and social cost of these complications to the community it is likely that the costs of more intensive treatment will be justifiable if treatment can be proved effective in preventing the complications.

How do the prudent clinician and patient act in the face of this uncertainty? There is general agreement that diabetes should be controlled as carefully as possible without producing disabling hypoglycaemia. The vigour with which normoglycaemia is pursued will depend on the rapport between patient and advisors, the degree of insight shown by the patient, the brittleness of the diabetes, the need to avoid hypoglycaemia and the conclusion reached from a study of the evidence outlined above.

Care of the foot

Within 10 years of the discovery of insulin, special measures were instituted to care for the feet of diabetic patients. It was demonstrated subsequently that the provision of 'a foot room' in a diabetic clinic had reduced the number of patients requiring admission to hospital, the number of amputations and the mortality (Brandaleone et al 1937). Care of the feet takes place at three levels:

1. The patient must take routine measures to care for his or her feet.

2. Early lesions require expert care either from a podiatrist or a doctor experienced in the care of these patients.

3. Advanced lesions require specialist surgical care.

The first two phases are the subject of this section. Detailed management of advanced lesions is given in Chapter 10.

Organization of care

The way in which care is organized will vary between different health care systems. At one extreme those involved in the management of these patients will act independently. The alternative model is for all concerned to provide a unified service involving multiple disciplines. Edmonds et al (1986) have provided good evidence of the results which can be obtained using such a clinic. Whichever model is adopted, good communication between all those involved is an essential component. This must include those outside hospital (the patient, family members involved in caring for the patient, visiting nurses, podiatrists and general medical practitioners) and those practising predominantly in hospitals and health centres (podiatrists, specialist physicians, patient educators, surgeons, including vascular surgeons, and makers of prosthetics and footwear). It is my view that all those mentioned have a role to play in the management of these patients and that professional jealousies that impair collaboration act to the detriment of the patient and are to be deplored. At different times one or other of those involved will have the major responsibility. However, it must be remembered that these patients require lifelong care so that everyone involved in their care must have an adequate understanding of both short-term and long-term requirements.

In practical terms all attendants and the patient must be aware of the need for regular careful examination of the foot. This examination should include inspection for deformities of the toes, bunions, callosities, evidence of pressure areas, particularly on the sole of the foot or heel, and careful inspection between the toes for cracks in the skin or ulcers.

Role of the patient

The prevention of foot lesions requires the co-operation of the patient and it is likely that the better the patient is informed about the disease the more he or she will be able to take a responsible part in the management. In this regard, associations of diabetic patients have a very valuable role in providing a forum in which diabetics can learn from each other, and through which information can be distributed.

Education of the patient is an essential function of all those caring for diabetics. Many clinics supply a list of printed instructions; part of such a leaflet is shown in Figure 7.1. The guidance should be simple and straight-forward and include information about the following aspects.

General.   Diabetes may affect the nerves so that pain signals arising in the foot do not reach the brain. This means that the diabetic loses the warning signals produced by injury. The diabetic must therefore use the other senses, especially the eyes and hands to detect the earliest signs of injury or infection because if these are neglected serious problems may develop.

Daily inspection.   Diabetics should inspect their feet every day and seek advice if any swelling, cracks in the skin, redness or sores are present. If vision is impaired, someone with better eyesight should be asked to inspect the feet.

Protection of feet.   Patients should be advised never to walk barefoot and to avoid shoes or sandals which leave the toes exposed.

Shoes.   Leather shoes, although more expensive, are preferred because they conform more easily to the shape of the foot than shoes made from synthetic materials. They must not cause abnormal pressure on any part of the foot. Shoes which try to make the foot conform to the currently fashionable shape must be avoided.

Many patients experience problems when wearing new shoes. New shoes often cause pressure or friction on areas of the foot. This is particularly

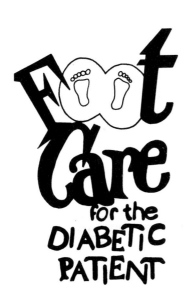

PROTECT
YOUR FEET BY . . . . .

AVOIDING EXPOSURE TO RAIN, COLD
AND EXCESSIVE SUNLIGHT

AND NEVER . . . . .

CUT CORNS AND CALLUSES WITH RAZOR-BLADE OR KNIFE

APPLY A HOT WATER BOTTLE, A HEATING PAD OR HOT WATER TO YOUR FEET

WEAR CUT OUT SHOES OR SANDALS

APPLY STRONG ANTISEPTIC OR CHEMICALS TO YOUR FEET

DON'T BE FOOT FOOLISH !

IT IS ESSENTIAL THAT YOU KEEP YOUR DIABETES UNDER GOOD CONTROL TO ENSURE GOOD FOOT CARE

DISCUSS ALL FOOT PROBLEMS PROMPTLY WITH YOUR PHYSICIAN OR PODIATRIST

Fig. 7.1   Part of the instruction leaflet issued by the Diabetic Clinic at the Royal Adelaide Hospital.

dangerous in a patient with neuropathy, because these stresses are not perceived as pain and severe damage may occur to the foot while the patient is unaware of any harm. When the shoes have been worn for several days they will adapt to the shape of the feet and damage to the skin of the foot is less likely to occur.

With new shoes a deliberate policy of 'breaking in' must be adopted. A new pair of shoes should not be worn for longer than two hours on the first occasion (see Fig. 6.2). At the end of that time the shoes should be removed and the feet inspected for any signs of redness or warmth which indicate that the area has been exposed to abnormal pressure or friction. Note that areas which have been subject to pressure may be pale initially.

The patients should develop the habit of inspecting and feeling the inside of each shoe for nails or foreign material before putting it on. No pair of shoes should be worn for longer than 4 or 5 hours if this can be avoided. Many patients keep a separate pair of shoes for wear at work. This means that footwear is changed at least twice each day.

Socks.   Woollen or heavy cotton socks or stockings should be chosen. For adequate cleanliness socks should be changed daily.

Bathing.   Feet should be washed daily using pure (non-medicated) soap, and dried carefully and gently, especially the area between the toes. Warm water may be used but the temperature of the water must be tested by hand to avoid scalding insensitive feet.

Toe nails.   Nails should be trimmed so that the distal edge is straight. The corners of the nails must not be rounded. A nail file or clipper may be used. If vision is impaired nails must only be treated by a podiatrist or other capable person.

Calluses and corns.   These must be treated with great care because they represent the response of the skin to pressure or friction. They may be rubbed with an emery board or pumice stone if the physician and podiatrist concur. No irritant chemicals may be used but emollient cream applied once or twice daily will soften the skin and allow easier removal of keratin. The cream should be rubbed into the skin and care taken that cream does not accumulate between the toes.

Heat.   A hot water bottle must never be placed against the skin of the feet.

No apology is necessary for repeating these simple instructions and no opportunity to reinforce them should be lost, because despite these well recognized objectives many problems arise. These include the ability of the attendant, physician, nurse or podiatrist, to communicate the importance of the message and the ability of the patient to comprehend the instructions and be motivated to follow them. Motivation is greatest soon after the diabetes has been diagnosed, later often a complacent attitude develops and the standard of care deteriorates as a result. Another opportunity for education is often provided by the first (hopefully minor) episode of infection or ulceration. The patient must have the physical capacity, e.g. eyesight and joint mobility to care for himself or herself and the social circumstances must be such that adequate care can be given. Unless all these elements — education, motivation and capacity to care for the feet, are present major difficulties will be encountered as can be seen by the frequency with which patients present with major lesions. Some problems result from minor accidents in well motivated patients but there are a large group of patients who lack insight or the capacity to care for their feet, and many intractable problems arise in this group.

MINOR LESIONS AND THEIR TREATMENT

The diabetic may suffer from all the foot conditions that a non diabetic may incur. Only those lesions of special importance to diabetics are discussed in this section. There is little epidemiological evidence regarding the frequency of these problems. In one population of diabetics in Finland there was a high incidence of minor abnormalities of the foot including ingrowing toenail (20%), other nail disorders (48%), hyperkeratosis (78%) and abnormal foot and toe posture (75%) (Ronnemaa et al 1988).

Role of the podiatrist

The podiatrist is an essential member of the team which cares for diabetics, taking a major responsibility for the provision of advice and support. The podiatrist fulfils several important roles.

Counselling. A visit to the podiatrist may be less daunting for the patients than making more visits to the doctor; patients often feel more relaxed and therefore more able to discuss their condition. The podiatrist should not lose any opportunity to advise the patient and particularly to warn against unsatisfactory footwear.

Treating minor lesions. There will be few communities where the available resources will allow all diabetics to receive care from a podiatrist. However, there are several categories of patient with a strong case for routine prophylactic care. These include patients with established arterial disease or neuropathy, particularly if there are additional medical or social factors such as visual impairment or impaired mobility, e.g. from arthritis.

A small area of hyper-keratosis, an ingrowing toe nail, or a small laceration may be trivial lesions in a foot with normal sensation and with a normal blood supply but to a diabetic with an ischaemic, neuropathic foot such lesions are potentially disastrous. These apparently minor incidents can be followed by rapidly-spreading infection or gangrene. The podiatrist attempts to reduce the progression of these lesions and advises the patient to consult the doctor as soon as this becomes necessary.

Performing foot surgery. This is an area of some controversy. The problem is to define the limits of the procedures which should be performed by the podiatrist. The boundaries are different in different communities and are set by local customs and/or laws. There is no doubt that many surgical procedures (defined as any procedure which requires incision of skin) can be performed safely on the feet of diabetic patients. However, there are substantial risks in performing surgery on a foot where neuropathy and ischaemia may be present and in a patient whose diabetes may be imperfectly controlled. It is my opinion that if these procedures are to be performed by a podiatrist, he or she should have demonstrated exceptional experience and judgement and should work closely with a group of physicians or surgeons who are accustomed to caring for diabetic patients. If there are signs of vascular insufficiency, surgical procedures should be carried out only in specialist centres.

Skin changes in diabetes

patients to look out for

A wide variety of dermatological conditions are recognized as occurring more commonly in diabetic patients (see Goodfield & Millard 1988 for review). The process of non-enzymic glycosylation (see p. 86) results in thickening of the collagen in the dermis, and 'browning' of collagen and keratin. There is also loss of elastic fibres. The result of these changes is that the skin is thick and less flexible, and this may make the skin more vulnerable to minor injury. The precise aetiology of these changes is uncertain although histological evidence of microangiopathy can be seen easily. These changes are not specific to diabetics but are more prominent in younger diabetic patients and in areas not normally exposed to sunlight.

Thick skin and stiff joints

These changes may occur in 30% of diabetics. They result in loss of extension of the fingers and ultimately a fixed flexion deformity. The joint stiffness rarely causes major disability. The changes are associated with other evidence of microvascular complications (Rosenbloom et al 1981).

Necrobiosis lipoidica diabeticorum

This lesion is common and occurs particularly on the lower leg. The lesions are plaques which may have a yellow centre and purple edge. They frequently form indolent superficial ulcers (Fig. 7.2). It is believed that these changes are a manifestation of microvascular disease in an area which even in normal subjects has a poor blood supply. As with other consequences of microvascular disease, there is no known specific treatment.

Lesions of the nails

These are discussed here because of their potential for causing serious problems. Like so many other aspects of the management of these patients the

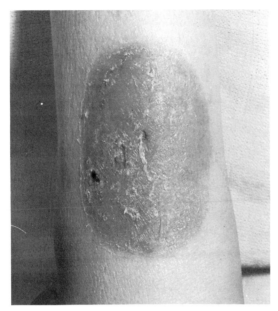

Fig. 7.2   Necrobiosis lipoidica diabeticorum of lower leg.

most important contribution to care is the prevention of problems. The instructions to the patient regarding care of the nails has been mentioned. If the nails are very thick or of the patient's eyesight or motor function are inadequate, care of the nails must be carried out by an attendant and this is usually the podiatrist.

Ingrowing toe nails

Infection or necrosis starting at the edge of an ingrowing toe nail has led to the amputation of many legs. A lesion which, in a normal foot, causes some discomfort and reduced mobility for a few days may, in an insensitive, ischaemic foot, be followed rapidly by spreading infection and necrosis. Any signs of infection around a toe nail must be regarded seriously and treated with rest and a full course of antibiotics. Evidence of necrosis (gangrene) is particularly sinister. The common cause of the lesion known as an ingrowing toe nail is frequently improper cutting of the nail with the corners of the nail cut proximally and not left square (Fig. 7.3a). A spur at the side of the nail breaks the epithelium adjacent to it and a chronic inflammatory reaction with granulation tissue formation is set up. This area provides a ready portal of entry for invasive organisms. The same result may follow the development of an excessively curved nail (Fig. 7.3b). The weight-bearing forces tend to drive the edges of the nail through the skin and the same risk of infection follows.

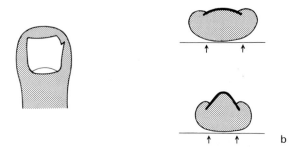

a   b

Fig. 7.3 (Left) The origin of an ingrowing toenail. The right hand corner of the nail has been cut back leaving a small spur projecting. As the nail grows this spur penetrates the skin. (Right) Problems with an excessively curved nail. In the normal toe (above) weight-bearing forces flatten the nail. With a very curved nail (below) the vertical forces tend to drive the edges of the nail into the soft tissues of the toe.

The most important part of management is prevention of the lesion by adequate podiatry and counselling. Early lesions may be treated by gently lifting the edge of the nail and placing a small rolled piece of cotton wool beneath it. Excision of a triangular piece from the leading edge of the nail may reduce the tendency to lateral growth. The podiatrist may remove a narrow piece from the lateral edge which should include the offending splinter of nail. The sulcus should be packed with cotton wool soaked in mild antiseptic. This dressing should be changed regularly and reviewed at weekly intervals during the initial stages to ensure that the lateral spur does not form again. If these measures fail to control the ingrowth and the ankle pulses are present, the nail should be removed.

Because of the danger of spreading necrosis which might lead to an amputation, removal of the nail from an ischaemic foot is very hazardous and should seldom be carried out and then only by a specialist. More extensive procedures such as removal of the nail bed are rarely necessary and are also specialist procedures in these patients.

Onychogryphosis

The development of thick curved nails (like sheep's horn) is very common in elderly patients. The danger is that the thick hard nail will cause pressure and necrosis at its edges or, more commonly, on an adjacent toe. The small lesion which results may, like an ingrown toe nail, be the focus through which infection enters and the sequelae may be just as disastrous. Preventative treatment is important. The overgrowth must be removed so that the remaining nail cannot cause pressure on neighbouring toes. This can be achieved by regular abrasion which should, at least initially, be carried out by an expert. It may be necessary to place small pads of cotton wool between the toes to avoid pressure from adjacent toes.

Fungal infections of skin and nails

These are reported to be more common in diabetics. The aetiology is uncertain but may result from trauma causing fissures in the nail bed which allow multiplication of the fungus. The presence of fungal and nail debris beneath the nail causes it to become thick and opaque. There may be a history of loss and regrowth of the nail. Long-term antibiotic therapy may be used but the infection frequently recurs following cessation. The best treatment is the regular removal of the abnormal nail tissue.

Fungal infections of the skin are indicated by itch, redness and desquamation, particularly in moist areas between the toes where the skin appears white and macerated. The condition is treated by careful drying of the skin and the application of topical antifungal agents.

Increased keratin formation

This is a normal response to increased pressure and friction on the skin and in normal feet there are areas where the keratin layer is thicker than in others. The presence of a localized increase in keratin should be regarded as indicating abnormal forces on the foot, rather than an abnormal propensity in the diabetic to form keratin. The common sites involved are the sole of the foot in the region of the metatarsal heads, the lateral side of the fifth metatarsal base and the medial side of both the head of the first metatarsal and the region of the interphalangeal joint of the great toe. If the toes are clawed, friction on the inside of the shoe may cause callus formation over the proximal interphalangeal joint. A distinction is often made between a corn which forms over a non-weight-bearing bony prominence and callus which forms over weight-bearing surfaces. A corn may be a more sharply circumscribed lesion and usually has a core which may cause tenderness. However, histologically the lesions are similar and they both arise from abnormal pressure or friction forces, so a rigid distinction between them seems artificial.

In the first instance, treatment is directed to removing the sources of trauma by the provision of adequate footwear and the local removal of hyperkeratoses. The role of the podiatrist in advising the patient regarding footwear has already been mentioned and this is the first and most important line of treatment. The callus may be removed by excision with a scalpel or by abrasion with emery boards or rotating burr (like a dentist's drill). The patient should be seen at regular intervals until the overgrowth of keratin has been controlled. Modification of footwear is often required. Long-term treatment may be necessary because the predisposing cause, e.g. an underlying exostosis, may remain. Chemical keratolytic agents should not be used and the patient must be discouraged from self-treatment with these materials because, if neuropathy is present, chemical damage to the skin may occur and not be recognized by the patient.

If providing adequate shoes does not give sufficient relief from the hyperkeratosis, various methods for the relief of pressure may be tried. Simple but effective measures include keeping toes apart with small pieces of cotton wool, and adhesive felt rings placed around the margins of a corn. Pads and plasters of various shapes may be used to relieve the pressure on the affected area by transferring it to adjacent areas. These may be purchased ready-made or cut to the desired pattern by the podiatrist. Great care must be taken that no new areas are endangered by these manoeuvres. More difficult and extensive lesions may require more elaborate appliances (see below). Operative treatment to remove underlying bony prominences must never be undertaken unless it is certain that the blood supply to the foot is normal. These procedures have very little place in the management of middle-aged diabetics.

Ulcers on toes

The commonest site for an ulcer is over the dorsum of the interphalangeal joint in a patient with clawed toes. In these cases any device which reduces the depth of the shoe must be removed because the definitive treatment of these lesions is relief of pressure or friction. Once adequate depth has been provided in the footwear the ulcer can be expected to heal. Ulcers of the tips of the toes (see Fig 8.5) which occur at an earlier stage of clawing are usually self-curing: as the deformity increases the pressure on the affected area decreases. Interdigital ulcers are usually caused by pressure from an adjacent toe nail and are treated by trimming the nail and keeping the toes apart with small cotton wool dressings or foam-rubber pads. These apparently minor lesions may cause serious problems in ischaemic feet and are discussed in more detail in Chapter 8.

Plantar ulcers

If an ulcer develops during a period of observation it means that, for whatever reason, the preventative measures have failed. The ulcer has developed because the skin has been exposed to excessive stresses which have not been adequately controlled. A much more serious phase of the disease begins because there is now, in addition to the chances of continuing necrosis, a portal of entry for bacteria which may lead to the development of infection with more tissue destruction. A detailed assessment of the situation by physician and podiatrist must be undertaken as described in Chapter 9. Many ulcers may continue to be managed in outpatients although much closer supervision will be needed.

The first sign that an ulcer has developed is the presence of some blood pigment in an area of thick callus. The floor of the ulcer may not be visible but the blood is a sure indication that the skin beneath has broken. As the callus is trimmed away, evidence of cavitation or necrosis is seen and finally the extent of the ulcer can be demonstrated. After passing the soft, soggy callus, an area of granulation tissue that forms the floor of the ulcer can be seen. The keratin should be removed until the white callus has been removed and soft pink skin can be seen all around the ulcer. A large disposable scalpel blade is an appropriate instrument for this task. The process should be repeated at regular intervals (e.g. fortnightly) until the build-up of callus is controlled.

After cleaning with saline, the ulcer should be covered with a piece of dry gauze which can be changed daily. Gauze soaked in a mild antiseptic, e.g. povidone iodine complex 1%, may be used.

These steps may be continued provided that the ulcer does not enlarge or signs of infection occur (p. 120). Enlargement is an indication for detailed assessment which may include tests of the blood supply and examination (e.g. X-ray and probing of the ulcer), to see if deeper structures have become involved. Infection is an indication for urgent admission to hospital and antibiotic therapy.

Relieving the pressure on the ulcerated area is the only way of allowing the ulcer to heal. This simple aim may be very difficult to achieve. The patient feels no pain and is able to walk normally so it is often difficult to convince him or her that a major alteration in his lifestyle may be needed. Rest in bed is the ideal way of reducing the load and allowing the ulcer to heal. However this is usually not possible on economic grounds from the view either of the patient or of the hospital system.

There are three methods which may be used to allow the patient to walk while healing is occurring, to protect the foot after healing of ulcers or amputation or to minimize damage in a persisting ulcer: insoles, shoes and plaster casts.

FOOTWEAR AND PROSTHETICS

Insoles

Appropriately designed insoles may relieve the pressure sufficiently so that healing can occur while the patient remains ambulatory. The chances of healing are increased if the patient can temporarily decrease the amount of walking, for example, by a period of rest in the afternoon.

Appliances that reduce the space available within the shoe must be used with extreme caution. A pad beneath the metatarsal heads may have some place in reducing the deformity of clawed toes, but it must only be used if the metatarsophalangeal and interphalangeal joints are still mobile. If the joints are stiff, the appliance will not reduce the deformity and will increase the damage by causing pressure between the dorsum of the interphalangeal joints and the shoe. Evidence of increased pressure such as hyperkeratosis or reddening must be sought very carefully if this device is used.

Insoles are especially useful in patients whose feet have been deformed by operation or who have planter ulcers. They may be used to protect exposed toes or to relieve pressure on particular areas of the foot. The polyethylene plastic, Plastazote, is a suitable material. It differs from a sponge in that the air pockets do not communicate with each other and it can be moulded when heated to 140°C. Figure 7.4 shows the design of a splint to lessen the pressure on the area of the second and third metatarsal heads. It is made from two pieces of material each 6 mm thick. An outline of the foot is traced on a sheet of Plastazote and the design of the second piece, shown shaded in the diagram, is drawn. The smaller piece is cut so that only one thickness of material lies beneath the area of the foot where relief from pressure is desired. This piece is placed in position and both put on a sheet of paper and heated in the oven. They have been adequately heated when they feel sticky to the palpating fingers. The two pieces will adhere when heated and the foot can be placed on the material as it cools but is still warm enough to mould. The foot is placed on the position originally outlined. A block of Plastazote approximately 20 mm thick should be placed on the floor beneath the splint. The edges of the splint can be trimmed to fit the shoe. If a mistake is made during this process, the Plastazote will regain its original shape after it is reheated in the oven. An alternative method is to use a single piece 12 mm thick. This will even out the distribution of load across the forefoot but probably does not produce the same reduction in load as the method described. Further sculpturing of the insole may be carried out with a knife or razor blade to produce greater relief from pressure in a desired area.

After the splint has been worn for several hours the shoes and stockings must be removed and the feet, especially the toes, inspected for signs of abnormal pressure. The splint may be washed weekly in warm water with mild detergent and can be expected to last 6–8 weeks of daily use. At the end of this time, it can be replaced or renewed by attaching a new piece of Plastazote beneath it. Figure 7.5 shows the effect of wearing this splint when tested on the apparatus described in Chapter 6. The reduction in load obtained, about 20% of the force under the designated area, is likely to be

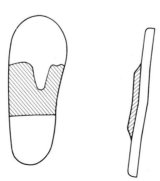

Fig. 7.4 Design of a Plastazote splint to relieve pressure on the heads of the second and third metatarsal bones.

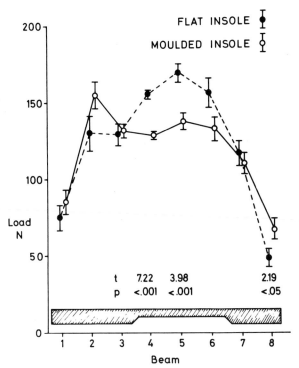

Fig. 7.5 Effect of wearing the splint shown in Fig. 7.4. There was a significant reduction in load in the area where the splint was thinnest (shown by the shaded area at the bottom of the figure).

great enough to make it clinically useful. Recently Boulton et al (1984) studied the effect of the visco-elastic polymer sorbothane placed between the foot and the load-sensitive area. Their method enabled them to study more clearly defined areas of the foot than in our original studies (see p. 83), and they were able to demonstrate significant reductions in load when walking on sorbothane, in many cases to normal levels (less than 10 kg/cm^2). This has the potential for major benefit to diabetic patients when used as insoles.

Plastazote may also be used to make a device which provides protection for exposed toes. Figure 7.6 shows a patient who developed an ulcer on the tip of the second toe which had been left exposed after removal of the great toe. A splint was constructed to protect the toes and the ulcer subsequently healed. The gap left by the removal of the great toe was filled by several pieces of Plastazote which were stuck together after heating their surfaces with a soldering iron. The piece covering the toes was similarly attached.

Plastazote has also been used to make sandals and shoes advocated for the treatment of patients with similar foot disorders particularly the deformities resulting from leprosy and rheumatoid arthritis.

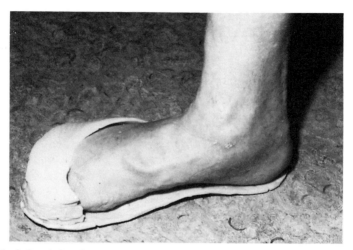

Fig. 7.6 Splint designed to protect the remaining toes after removal of the great toe. The toes are covered by a thin piece of Plastozote.

There are several other ways in which the problem of redistributing the load under the foot might be approached. One method uses the principle that water transmits pressure equally in all directions. Preliminary tests have shown that this method may be effective. Part of the sole of a shoe was cut away and a bag containing water was inserted. Testing of this device clearly showed that there was a reduction in the peak loads carried. The problem not yet solved is to contain the water in a material which is strong enough to withstand the repetitive forces produced by walking for a long period.

These devices may be of benefit to individual patients. Their design and fabrication requires much time and attention to detail but the potential rewards are great.

Shoes

In the section on advice to the patient it was pointed out that diabetics should never walk barefoot and should never wear any footwear that caused trauma to the feet. The design of the footwear depends on climate and culture, but protection and avoidance of injury are universal requirements. The routine instructions detailed (p. 94) can, if appropriately communicated and accepted, be very effective in reducing morbidity. However, it is possible to define several groups of patients who have a high risk of development or progression of ulcers and these groups of patients require more specialized care. They are:

1. Patients with feet deformed by neuropathic change, particularly where the deformity is a result of changes in the joints of the foot. Considerable deformity can be produced and this makes the wearing of

conventional shoes very difficult and unsafe. In other patients, clawing of the toes, resulting from denervation of the small muscles of the foot, sometimes produces a forefoot which can be safely fitted in a shoe only if the distance between the sole and upper is much greater than normal. This abnormality is sufficiently common that in many Western communities 'extra depth' shoes may be purchased off the shelf.

2. Patients with feet deformed as a result of operation. This may happen either because removal of a metatarsal head reduces the number of weight-bearing points from five to four, or because removal of a toe leaves neighbouring toes exposed. The possibility of removing these exposed digits is discussed in Chapter 10.

3. Patients with plantar ulcers. In some cases, after assessment as outlined in Chapter 9, it may be decided to treat the ulcer while allowing the patient to continue to walk. Patients who have recently healed plantar ulcers certainly require careful follow-up and many need modification of the footwear. There are several ways in which footwear can be modified to meet the changed requirements of these patients.

Custom-built shoes

The provision of custom-built shoes for many diabetics is beyond the financial resources of most communities and the craftsmen to make them are in short supply. Shoes are time-consuming and expensive to produce and there is a great potential for waste because the shape of the foot may be altered by operation a short time after the shoes are obtained. Nevertheless, for patients with grossly deformed feet the provision of special footwear is highly desirable. There may be ready-made shoes available that have enough extra depth between the sole and the upper to allow the insertion of an insole and provide space so clawed toes do not rub against the shoe. Extra depth to allow insertion of a 1 cm thick insole is often necessary. Specially made shoes must be made to enclose the foot comfortably. The appearance of the shoes must be as close as possible to that which is fashionable because shoes which are considered ugly by the patient may be discarded.

The effect of different patterns of shoes on the distribution of forces under the foot was studied by Bauman et al (1963) using transducers beneath the foot as described on page 84. They studied patients with neuropathy due to leprosy, and divided the subjects with anaesthetic feet into those with and without deformity. Those with deformity, which included the effects of repeated ulceration and loss of toes, were more closely related to the problem discussed here. The shoe which produced the greatest relief of load on the forefoot had two design features: a rigid sole, and a rocker placed behind the area of the metatarsal heads (Fig. 7.7). During the step-off phase (see p. 83), when the load is normally concentrated on the metatarsal heads, the effect of these modifications is to

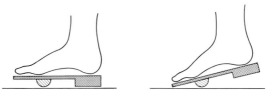

Fig. 7.7　Principles of a rocker shoe.

transfer part of the load to the area behind the metatarsal heads and away from the area which is most susceptible to the development of ulcers. Conventional shoes which are acceptable in appearance may be constructed incorporating these principles. The sole is made rigid by the insertion of a steel plate and the rocker bar may be added beneath the sole.

Plaster casts

Immobilization in a plaster cast is regularly used in third world countries to treat severely ulcerated feet in patients with diabetes or leprosy. The patient is able to continue walking while healing occurs and so does not need a hospital bed. This method should probably be used more frequently, although the excellent results obtained in communities where arterial disease is infrequent may not be easily obtainable in a Western community.

Like so many other situations in the management of these patients, this method requires meticulous care and rigorous attention to detail.

The technique used by Brand will be described. Small pieces of padding are applied to the anterior surface of the tibia, to the malleoli and dorsal surface of the ankle joint. A single plaster bandage is applied from the region of the metatarsal heads to the upper tibia and moulded to conform exactly to the contour of the leg and foot. If this is adequately achieved, there is no movement between limb and plaster, friction injuries will not occur and the forces during walking are evenly distributed over as wide an area as possible. When this bandage is almost dry, sufficient extra plaster is added to make the cast rigid and a rubber heel is added to allow weight bearing. The cast may be removed after 3 or 4 weeks and the progress of healing reviewed.

An alternative casting technique has been used by Pollard & Le Quesne (1983). They applied a conventional padded cast with good results. The amount of padding used and the exposure of the toes to allow changing of dressings on the ulcer distinguishes this technique from Brand's method.

There is no doubt that plaster casting is an effective method of treatment for patients with plantar ulcers, including some with extensive disease. However, my impression is that the technique is used infrequently in Western countries. Several colleagues in different countries have told me that they have seen occasional disastrous results, as a consequence of either undetected infection or the development of new pressure areas, particularly when the total contact cast has been used. The difficulties of the technique are largely related to the need for careful application of the plaster, remembering that the absence of pain sensation means that the patient will not complain of pain from developing plaster sores. Even when the ulcer is healed the problem is not over. The newly healed skin is very fragile and must be protected. The sources of external pressure which led to the development of the ulcer must be controlled and this often requires the combined attention of podiatrist, orthotist and shoemaker. Finally, and this is often the most difficult part, the patient must understand that preventative measures have to be continued for life.

REFERENCES

Bauman J H, Girling J P, Brand P W 1963 Plantar pressures and trophic ulceration. Journal of Bone and Joint Surgery 45B: 652–673
Boulton A J M, Franks C I, Betts R P, Duckworth T, Ward J D 1984 Reduction of abnormal foot pressures in diabetic neuropathy using a new polymer insole material. Diabetes Care 7: 42–46
Brandaleone H, Standard S, Ralli E P 1937 Prophylactic foot treatment in patients with diabetes mellitus. Annals of Surgery 105: 120–124
Brooks A P, Nairn I M, Baird J D 1980 Changes in glycosolated haemoglobin after poor control in insulin-dependent diabetics. British Medical Journal 281: 707–710
Cahill G F, Etzweiler D D, Freinkel N 1976 'Control' and diabetes. New England Journal of Medicine 294: 1004–1005
Edmonds M E, Blundell M P, Morris M E, Thomas E M, Cotton L T, Watkins P J 1986 Improved survival of the diabetic foot: the role of a specialised foot clinic. Quarterly Journal of Medicine 60: 763–771
Goldstein D E 1984 Is glycosylated hemoglobin clinically useful? New England Journal of Medicine 310: 384–385
Goodfield M J D, Millard L G 1988 The skin in diabetes. Diabetologia 31: 567–575
Koenig R G, Cerami A 1980 Haemoglobin A and diabetes mellitus. Annual Review of Medicine 31: 29–34
Nathan D M, Singer D E, Hurxthal D, Goodson J D 1984 The clinical information value of the glycosylated haemoglobin assay. New England Journal of Medicine 310: 341–346
Pollard J P, Le Quesne L P 1982 Method of healing diabetic forefoot ulcers. British Medical Journal 1: 436–437
Ronnemaa T, Knuts L-R, Liukkonen I 1988 Prevalence of foot problems and need for foot care in an unselected diabetic population. Diabetologia 31: 536A
Rosenbloom A L, Silverstein J H, Lezote D C, Richardson K, McCallum M 1981 Limited joint mobility in childhood diabetes mellitus indicates increased risk of microvascular disease. New England Journal of Medicine 305: 191–194
Siperstein M D, Foster D W, Knowles H C, Levine R, Madison L L, Ruth J 1977 Control of blood glucose and diabetic vascular disease. New England Journal of Medicine 296: 1060–1063
Skyler J S 1989 Issues, controversies and directions in diabetes care. In: Larkins R G, Zimmet P, Chisholm D J (eds) Diabetes 1988. Exerpta Medica, Amsterdam p 793–802
Tchobroutsky G 1978 Relation of diabetic control to development of microvascular complications. Diabetologia 15: 143–152

8. Clinical features of major lesions

Despite the efforts of patient and attendants, major lesions may develop. It is the purpose of this chapter to describe the ways in which these patients present. All too often, patients come for treatment with a foot which has been swollen and discharging for days or weeks. These patients will usually notice, if they test their urine, that glycosuria has increased. At this stage admission to hospital is necessary and will probably be followed by one or more operations, a prolonged period of immobility and possible loss of a major part of the foot or limb. Many minor lesions can be managed or prevented from extending by provision of adequate footwear and careful podiatry (Ch. 7).

THE VULNERABLE FOOT

A foot in which arterial disease, neuropathy or both are present is liable to develop major complications. The effects of arterial disease and neuropathy have been described in Chapters 3 and 4 respectively, and the detailed presenting features are given below. However, it is helpful to summarize the clinical findings in a foot in which the conditions for the development of a major lesion exist. Detailed assessment is discussed in Chapter 9.

Evidence of ischaemia:

History of intermittent claudication or rest pain
Coldness of the foot
Absence of ankle pulses
Dependent rubor.

(Standard textbooks often provide a longer list of features but those given here will enable adequate assessment to be made.)

Evidence of neuropathy:

Clawing of the toes
Callus over pressure areas

Deformity due to neuropathic changes in joints
The foot feels dry and also warm if the blood supply is sufficient
Loss of light touch and pain (pin prick) sensation on the toes and
foot. In more severe cases this sensory loss may extend to the calf
Loss of perception of vibration on the foot, at the ankle and perhaps
at the knee
Absence of ankle tendon reflexes and perhaps patellar tendon reflexes.

Evidence of previous episodes:

Any patient who has had an ulcer or amputation of a toe or part of
the foot has a high risk of developing further problems.

A patient with one or more of these groups of features must be very
carefully supervized and may need special footwear as described in Chapter
7. Many patients are able to avoid the development of major lesions but it
is from this population that the difficult problems of assessment and
management will occur.

The following sections describe the common modes of presentation of
major lesions of the foot. This listing is not exclusive and represents a
simplification because combinations of lesions frequently occur. However it
is helpful to consider these principal ways in which the patients present.

THE ACUTE FOOT

Some diabetics present with acute problems, which may threaten the
survival of the foot.

Infection

This mode of presentation is most common in developing countries.
The factors responsible for these presentations have been summarized by
Mustapha & Ngan (1989). They include a high prevalence of undetected
diabetes and a high incidence of neuropathy in diabetic patients. To these
must be added social and cultural factors and, in many cases, limited access
to skilled medical care.

Infection in a neuropathic foot is the dominant factor in these presentations.
There may or may not have been an area of damaged skin before the onset
of the infection. The commonest presentation is of a deep infection in a
neuropathic foot (see p. 120). These patients must be treated urgently to:

1. Control diabetes with insulin and intravenous fluids
2. Limit the spread of infection by antibiotic therapy
3. Drain the infection. See Chapter 10.

Ischaemia

Acute arterial occlusion may result from embolism to the arteries of the leg or thrombosis occurring on a diseased artery wall (see p. 13). The presenting features are sudden onset of pain, pallor and coldness of the foot. There may be paraesthesiae and numbness which spreads proximally and muscle pain and weakness. The principles of management are identical in diabetics and non-diabetics and include heparin, thrombolytic therapy and operation (embolectomy and/or thrombectomy and/or bypass). For detailed plans of management, texts on vascular surgery should be consulted. There is a significant risk to both life and limb in these patients who almost all have severe cardiovascular disease.

TYPES OF LESIONS

Lesions can be conveniently classified on their macroscopic appearance as being ulcers, gangrene or infection. In many cases two or three processes may coexist. It is important not to make too rigid the distinction between ulcers and gangrene. An ulcer, which is defined as a break in an epithelial surface, may contain areas of necrosis or gangrene. A gangrenous toe may separate leaving an ulcer, the floor of which is healthy granulation tissue. It is however, conventional to classify the lesions with a label that reflects the major changes in the area.

Gangrene

Gangrene of toe(s)

Gangrene of the toe often starts from a minor injury, e.g. while cutting the toe nail, although in many cases the initial lesion is not recognized. The wound fails to heal, the skin edges become black and the gangrene extends to involve the whole toe. Adjacent toes may also become gangrenous. There is often a clear demarcation between living and dead tissues (dry gangrene), although the gangrene may gradually progress to involve the foot (Fig. 8.1). There is frequently a surrounding area of cellulitis of variable extent.

The lesion may arise in two ways:

Atherosclerotic occlusion of arteries. These occlusions occur particularly in the thigh and/or calf (see p. 17). The features of chronic ischaemia of the foot are present: cool foot, absent pulses and dependent rubor. Ischaemic rest pain is present if there is not severe neuropathy. The pain may have preceded the development of gangrene. These patients require arterial surgery to improve the blood supply to the foot and allow healing to occur.

Occlusion of digital arteries. The implication is that the blood supply to the remainder of the foot is sufficient for the survival of the foot. The foot

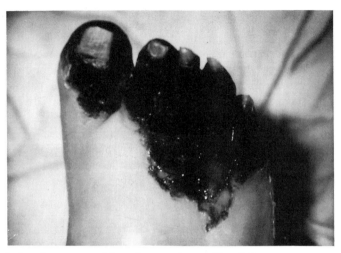

Fig. 8.1 Ischaemic gangrene of foot. (Same patient as Fig. 10.3).

is warm and ankle pulses may be palpable. There are features of neuropathy, especially reduced perception of pain. In these cases healing can be expected to follow local amputation. Digital artery occlusion may occur as a result of damage to the vessel wall by spreading infection following minor injury. This outcome is potentiated if there is arterial disease involving the digital and metatarsal arteries (see p. 22).

Gangrenous patches

Areas of gangrene may occur on parts of the foot that are exposed to pressure. The common sites are the heel, the malleoli and the areas of the first metatarsal head medially, and the base of the fifth metatarsal. They may vary from a few millimetres to several centimetres in diameter (Figs. 8.2, 8.3). They typically occur in bedridden patients who have severe atherosclerosis but neuropathy is frequently present so the lesions do not cause pain. They often remain about the same size and sometimes heal slowly. They sometimes develop during treatment for some other condition (Fig. 8.4), such as a lesion of the other foot. Meticulous nursing care is essential to prevent their occurrence.

Small areas of gangrene may also occur on parts of the foot not subject to pressure because of embolism of atheromatous debris. Small infarcts in the skin result. There are usually multiple areas 2–3 mm in diameter in several parts of the toes and foot (Fig. 8.5). These are a purple-blue colour and do not blanch on pressure. They are usually painful and may heal beneath a small scab or eschar which forms on the skin. These lesions are atherosclerotic in origin and not specific to diabetics. The large arteries are usually patent (otherwise the emboli would not have reached the skin).

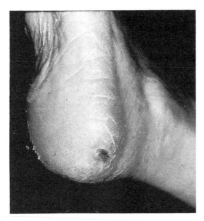

Fig. 8.2 Small area of gangrene in heel. This probably started in a crack in the normal thick keratin of the heel.

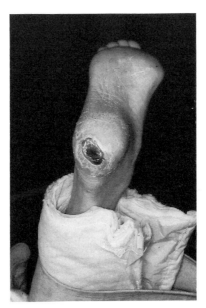

Fig. 8.3 Large area of gangrene of the heel. This is commonly seen in bedridden patients and results from prolonged pressure on the area. The necrosis extends to the calcaneum and major amputation is necessary in many cases.

The debris may be thrombus arising from an aneurysm, e.g. of the aorta or popliteal artery or debris from an atherosclerotic plaque in any proximal artery. Occasionally the areas of necrosis are so large that amputation of a toe is required.

Gangrenous patches may form in the interdigital clefts. The initiating factor may be pressure from adjacent toes. They are usually painful but

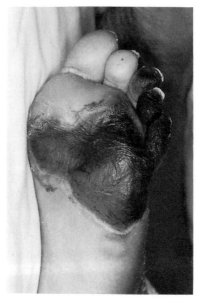

Fig. 8.4 Area of gangrene in the sole of the foot in a patient with a fracture of the shaft of the femur. The necrosis resulted from pressure from an appliance used to prevent foot drop.

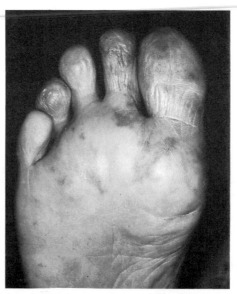

Fig. 8.5 Areas of ischaemic skin from occlusion of small vessels with atheromatous debris. (This patient was not diabetic).

easy to overlook because gentle separation of the toes is essential to see the lesions. They are frequently associated with severe ischaemia. They are difficult to manage because their proximal position means that infection may spread directly to the deep plantar spaces.

Bullous lesions are often superficial blisters that heal rapidly but deeper lesions which result in areas of skin necrosis can occur (Hadden & Allen 1969).

Gangrene with infection

Dead tissue is always contaminated with bacteria. However, in most patients with gangrene as described above, invasive infection does not occur. In some situations gangrene and invasive infection occur together.

Spreading atherosclerotic gangrene. This begins as outlined in the previous section. If infection follows, it may spread through tissue which, because of a poor blood supply, is unable to confine the process so that further necrosis occurs (wet gangrene). This type of gangrene is a threat to life because spreading anaerobic cellulitis may follow. Infection is the dangerous outcome of conservative treatment of gangrene although such a policy is often justified by the age and general condition of the patient. Wet gangrene occurs in non-diabetics as well as in diabetics.

Gangrene in a well vascularized foot (Fig. 8.6). This is one of the

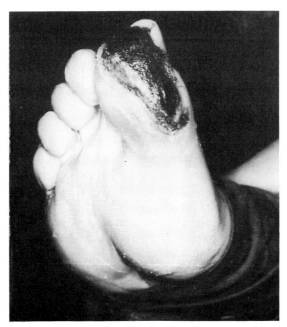

Fig. 8.6   Gangrene in a well vascularized foot. In this case gangrene followed wearing a new pair of shoes. Both ankle pulses were present.

characteristic lesions in diabetics and is sometimes labelled 'diabetic gangrene'. It is distinguished from the gangrene described above because it develops rapidly and is almost painless because of severe neuropathy. It may start in a manner identical to atherosclerotic gangrene, e.g. from a minor wound on a toe. Necrosis may extend because the infection causes thrombosis of digital vessels. Signs of deep infection in the foot are usually present, the foot is warm and ankle pulses can be felt if they are not masked by oedema. Often attention is drawn to the foot by the smell from the infected tissue rather than by pain. The necrosis may involve extensive areas, e.g. several toes and the adjacent part of the foot. There may be severe systemic effects including loss of control of diabetes, ketosis and septicaemia. It should be remembered that the blood supply to the foot is normal in most of these patients and healing will follow adequate drainage.

Anaerobic cellulitis. See page 123.

Ulcers

Plantar ulcers

Plantar ulcer is the characteristic neuropathic foot lesion of the diabetic. Synonyms include trophic or penetrating ulcer and mal perforans. They are typically painless and occur over areas that normally carry weight or which, because of structural changes, have come to carry excessive weight. The mechanisms by which they develop have been discussed in Chapter 6 (p. 88). The earliest change is an area of hyperkeratosis often over a metatarsal head. The keratin may be several millimetres thick at its centre. If uncontrolled, a small area of dark staining eventually appears in the keratin. This material, which is altered blood, indicates that the epithelium beneath has been breached. If the excess keratin is pared away a small ulcer will be found. At this stage the ulcer is often no more than a linear split in the skin. If the area of pressure is unrelieved, the ulcer will enlarge, often reaching 1–2 cm in diameter (Fig. 8.7). As the ulcer enlarges it involves the deeper tissues of the foot, progressively involving aponeurosis, tendon sheath and bone. Infection may occur at any stage and may spread along tendon sheaths or other planes opened up by the extension of the ulcer. In a deformed foot, e.g. following neuropathic degeneration of the tarsal joints, ulcers may develop over the resulting bony prominences (see p. 86). These ulcers are notoriously resistant to treatment if walking continues.

Signs of neuropathy are detectable; diminution or absence of the perception of pain is almost always present. The circulation to the foot may range from normal to severely impaired but, characteristically, it is good enough to allow healing if the loads which caused the ulcer are reduced. The complications of these ulcers are progressive tissue necrosis and infection. The non-operative management of these ulcers has been discussed in the previous chapter (p. 103). The indications for, and details of, operative treatment are given in Chapter 10.

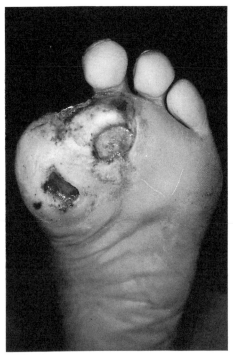

Fig. 8.7   Two ulcers on the sole of the foot. Note thick, white hyperkeratotic areas.

Ulcers of the toes

The commonest site for an ulcer of the toe is on the dorsum of the proximal interphalangeal joint of a clawed toe. These toes, because they are raised dorsally beyond the plane of the foot, are often rubbed by the inside of the shoe. Hyperkeratosis or inflammation may precede the breakdown of the skin and the development of a small ulcer. If the blood supply to the foot is impaired, the ulcer may initiate the development of gangrene as outlined above. If infection becomes established in the ulcer, it may result in gangrene or spread to the deep tissues of the foot.

Ulcers may develop on the tips of the toes (Fig. 8.8). This occurs during the early stages of clawing when the tips of the toes still make contact with the ground.

Pressure from adjacent toes or toe nails may also cause ulcers. They occur commonly on the lateral side of the third or fourth toes due to pressure from the fourth or fifth toe respectively. These ulcers are usually painless but they may be quite deep and involve an underlying interphalangeal joint. In addition, they present a portal of entry for infection.

The medial side of the interphalangeal joint of the great toe frequently develops ulcers analogous to the plantar ulcers described above. This lesion reflects disordered forefoot function and may be associated with hallux

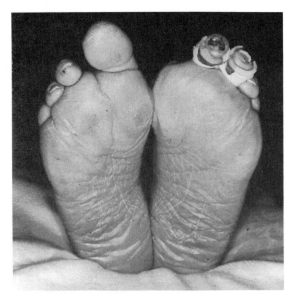

Fig. 8.8 Ulcers on tips of clawed toes.

rigidus which limits extension of the first metatarsophalangeal joint. The ulcer frequently extends to the interphalangeal joint which becomes infected.

Infection

The diabetic is liable to the whole range of infections that affect non-diabetics. These include non-specific bacterial infections, as well as specific mycotic infections which are particularly common in tropical climates. The diagnosis of infection is made difficult because of the loss of one of the cardinal symptoms of infection, pain. Moreover, the systemic sign of sepsis may appear late in the process. Unexplained hyperglycaemia is an important sign.

Deep infection

Because of the absence of pain, the presence and extent of infections is often underestimated. Although the severe throbbing pain associated with an abscess is not present, there is often a dull ache or burning or tingling sensation reported. There is often pus discharging through a sinus or ulcer which preceded the infection. The discharge of pus can be produced by pressure over the mid part of the sole or by moving an infected joint (Fig. 8.9). The most important signs are swelling and redness (Fig. 8.10), which may be seen in the dorsum of the web spaces of the foot because many of the lymphatics from the superficial tissues drain in this direction. Swelling of the toes may also be a useful sign. However the most characteristic sign is separation of the toes due to diffuse oedema of the deep tissues of the foot, and this almost always means that there is pus deep in the foot. The thickness of the plantar fascia masks swelling of the anterior part of the sole of the foot, but swelling and redness may be seen inferior and posterior to the medial malleolus. This is because the infection commonly tracks along the flexor tendon sheaths which pass behind the medial malleolus. These sheaths also provide the route by which infection may spread into the lower part of the leg. Any of these signs indicate that the patient should be admitted to hospital.

The amount of necrosis visible varies widely. At one extreme there may be only a small puncture wound (Fig. 8.10). More usually there is evidence of plantar ulceration or ulceration overlying a joint (Fig. 8.9). Sometimes there will be major areas of necrosis present as described on page 157. The important point about all these patients is to recognize that deep infection is present and, in virtually every case, will require surgical drainage. Failure to recognize these features may result in loss of the foot because, as long as deep infection remains undrained, necrosis in the deep tissues of the foot will continue and progress.

A localized abscess may also form on the dorsum of the foot. Infection here follows a lesion on a toe. Swelling is very common in this site because the subcutaneous tissue is relatively loose and the lymphatics run through the area. The sign of fluctuation may be difficult to detect because the pus may be deep to the extensor tendons. A small collection of pus is frequently found here when deep infections of the sole of the foot are being drained, e.g. by a ray amputation (see p. 165). In the most severe cases, there will be swelling and redness in the calf, indicating that the infection has spread to that region. Once this stage has been reached it is likely that the foot will be lost.

In patients with infection of the foot, a plain radiograph may show gas in the tissues. This is an important sign of severe infection but does not necessarily indicate clostridial cellulitis (see below). A number of bacteria, including anaerobic streptococci, Proteus species, *Escherischia coli*, klebsiella, enterobacter and enterococci, may form gas in the tissues.

Anaerobic infections

These are very dangerous because of the rapidity with which they spread and cause a systemic infection. Ischaemia of the tissues is an important predisposing factor. They may occur in any foot in which the skin has been broken but they are particularly likely to occur following surgery, e.g. local amputation. Fortunately most of the infections with anaerobic bacteria, e.g. bacteroides species, remain localized. There are two forms of spreading anaerobic infection.

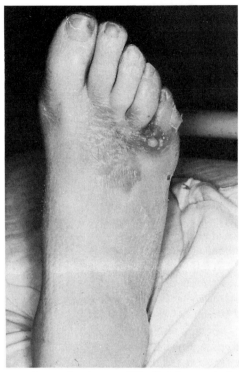

Fig. 8.9 Infection presenting on the dorsum of the foot from a plantar ulcer involving the fifth metatarsophalangeal joint. When the fifth toe was moved, pus exuded from the white area at the base of the toe.

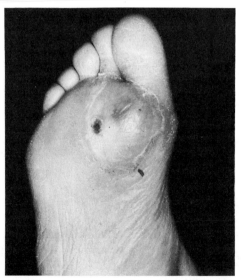

Fig. 8.10 Cellulitis in the foot due to an unnoticed drawing pin through the sole of the shoe. An area of redness extends to the base of the great toe. Drainage was not required.

Clostridial. The infection is identical to that occurring in non-diabetics. The classical form is a spreading myositis, in which the patient has evidence of severe generalized infection, with a high fever and leucocytosis. Less often there may be a spreading subcutaneous infection, in which gas is present but where the skin appears relatively healthy until late in the disease. Gram-positive spore-forming bacilli will be seen in a smear from the affected tissue and sometimes, shortly before death, in a smear from the peripheral blood.

Non-Clostridial. The features of non-clostridial gas gangrene in diabetics have been described by Bird et al (1977). They include insidious onset, absence of pain and the late appearance of skin necrosis and crepitus.

NEUROPATHIC JOINT DEGENERATION (Charcot's joints)

A non-infective joint degeneration may occur in patients with denervated joints. These changes were first described by Charcot in 1868 in a patient with locomotor ataxia (tabes dorsalis). They have since been described in many conditions in which there is loss of sensory innervation of joints. In diabetics, joints of the lower limb are predominantly affected. Those usually involved are the metatarsophalangeal joints and the joints between the tarsal and metatarsal bones. Occasionally the ankle and knee joints are affected and there have been reports of involvement of the upper limb and spine.

The mechanism postulated for these changes is that the joints become damaged by repetitive strain injuries which are not recognized because of neuropathy. Ligamentous laxity is followed by the formation of fragments of bone and cartilage which become enclosed in proliferated synovial membrane. It is presumed that these fragments are worn off the bones as a consequence of the excessive range of movement allowed by the lax ligaments. These fragments are absorbed and the bones become sclerotic as the acute process subsides. Severe deformity may occur in weight-bearing joints. An adequate blood supply is essential to allow the acute inflammatory and reactive changes which occur. Arteriovenous shunting (p. 28) has been considered to be an aetiological factor.

Patients commonly present with a history of weeks or months of swelling, redness and sometimes pain in the affected area. Most have had diabetes for more than 10 years. These lesions are usually seen in middle-aged patients but are sometimes seen in patients younger than 30. There are conflicting accounts of the importance of poor diabetic control as a predisposing factor but evidence of neuropathy is always present.

The radiological appearances vary with the area involved. Characteristic features include both destructive and hypertrophic changes. There is loss of joint space, and fragmentation and absorption of subchondral bone. Large osteophytes form at the joint margins and these may fracture. The appearances are of severe disorganization of the joint. In the diabetic, the tarsal bones are most often affected by this process and the resulting appearances may suggest that one of the bones, e.g. the navicular, has almost completely disappeared. The appearances are different when the distal parts of the metatarsal bones or the phalanges are affected and these changes are sometimes described as 'atrophic'. There is destruction of the epiphyseal bone of the metatarsal heads and phalanges (Figs. 8.11–8.13). The shafts of the bones may be thinned with the result that the metatarsal shaft tapers to a pointed end. Neuropathic changes may be difficult to distinguish from those associated with infection (see p. 132). If there is an ulcer beneath an affected joint, infection of the joint should be assumed. In addition, if there is clinical evidence of infection in the foot, the joint is likely to be involved. Healing of the foot may occur in the absence of acute infection but should healing not occur, gentle probing of the ulcer will usually reveal a communication with the underlying bone. In these circumstances the infected bone should be excised (see Ch. 10).

Progressive deformity may occur following subsidence of the acute reaction. There may be increasing deformity, crepitus and multiple loose bodies around the joint. If the tarsal joints are involved (Figs. 8.13–.15) there may be collapse of the longitudinal arch and bony prominence in the region of the navicular or cuboid bones. The skin over this area becomes weight bearing ('rocker foot'). Intractible ulceration is a frequent outcome (Fig. 8.14).

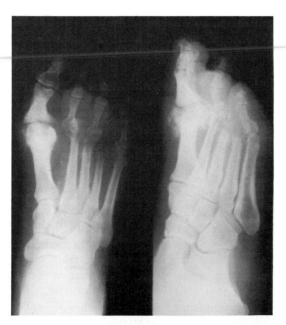

Fig. 8.11 Destruction and new bone formation of the first metatarsophalangeal joint. Destruction of the 2nd–4th metatarsophalangeal joints. Apparent loss of 4th toe. Bones of metatarsals and tarsal bones appear normal. (Patient of Mr J. H. Miller Vascular Surgeon, Royal Adelaide Hospital, South Australia).

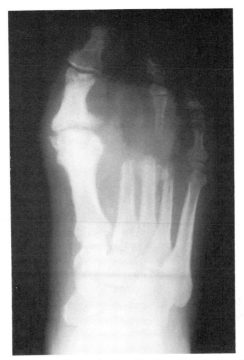

Fig. 8.12   The same patient as Fig. 8.11, six weeks later. Resolution of changes in 1st metatarsophalangeal joint. Apparent loss of 2nd and 4th toes. Subluxation of head of 3rd metatarsal.

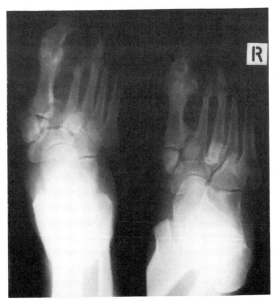

Fig. 8.13   The same patient as Fig. 8.11, seven months after presentation. Chronic changes in 1st metatarsophalangeal joint. Atrophic changes in 2nd and 4th metatarsals. Sclerosis of cunieform bones. Subluxation of base of metatarsals.

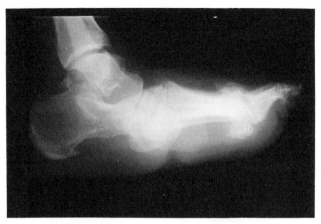

Fig. 8.14 Lateral view of the foot sham in Figs. 8.11–8.13. 'Rocker-foot' with plantar protrusion of cuboid. Soft tissue shadow of ulcer can be seen.

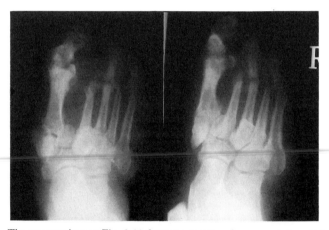

Fig. 8.15 The same patient as Fig. 8.11 fourteen months after presentation. Sclerosis and new bone in region of bone in first metatarsal and distal part of navicular. Subluxation of base of metatarsals.

There is no established treatment to halt this degenerative process. It is suggested that avoidance of weight bearing or rigid immobilization lessens the deformity but in many patients deformity has developed by the time of presentation. The management of these feet places a great strain on the resources of both podiatrist and bootmaker. Once ulcers occur, spontaneous healing is unlikely and recurrent ulceration frequently follows short periods of healing.

The discussion has concentrated on the presentation of major foot lesions almost all of which will require treatment as an in-patient in hospital. Details of the assessment of the patients are given in Chapter 9 and treatment in Chapter 10.

REFERENCES

Bird D, Giddings A E B, Jones S M 1977 Non-clostridial gas gangrene in the diabetic lower limb. Diabetologia 13: 373–376
Hadden D R, Allen G E 1969 Bullous lesions of the feet of diabetic patients. Diabetologia 5: 422
Mustapha B E, Ngan A 1989 The foot at risk, problems in developing countries. In: Larkins R G, Zimmet P, Chisholm D J (eds) Diabetes 1988. Exerpta Medica, Amsterdam p 1051–6

9. Assessment of the patient with a foot lesion

Vascular disease and neuropathy set the scene for the development of complications. Infection, which may be so important in causing tissue damage, follows some breach in the skin which either passes unrecognized due to neuropathy or fails to heal because of an impaired arterial supply. In considering the development of foot lesions, arterial disease and neuropathy must be regarded as developing and progressing independently, despite the possible role of arterial disease as a cause of neuropathy. This means that patients are encountered with all possible combinations: from extensive arterial disease with no detectable neuropathy, to severe neuropathy with no detectable arterial disease. Most commonly, both are present and the aim of assessment is to determine the contribution made by each.

Some patients present with an infected foot which is a serious threat to life and limb (see p. 112). However, a gangrenous or ulcerated limb is not an immediate threat to life unless a severe infection supervenes. This means that in most cases there is time to make a careful assessment of both the general condition of the patient and the state of the foot.

The development of a serious foot lesion is a major event in the natural history of diabetes and provides an opportunity for a detailed assessment of the patient, particularly with regard to the development of diabetic complications. After this assessment and the treatment of life-threatening complications, the likely outcome of the episode must be considered. The two extreme outcomes are: the lesion will heal, or that a major amputation will be needed. In between are the possibilities that reconstructive surgery or a minor amputation may be necessary. Firm decisions cannot be made before a detailed review has been made of the general and local condition.

Most patients can be successfully assessed by standard clinical techniques and simple laboratory tests. There is no doubt, however, that the difficulties of making precise assessments cause mistakes to be made. The recent growth of interest in this subject has resulted in the application of a variety of tests to study these patients. Our understanding of the pathophysiology of these disorders has been increased as a result and some of the information has been of value in the management of the patients. A variety of methods of greater or lesser complexity is available to provide additional information and the value and limitations of these measurements will be discussed.

GENERAL ASSESSMENT

Control of diabetes

The state of diabetic control must be assessed. The urine is examined for sugar and ketones and the blood glucose level determined. The problems of assessing the medium to long-term control of diabetes have been discussed on page 91. The urgency of regaining control depends on the severity of the foot lesion but in more severe cases it is necessary to substitute regular insulin injections for the patient's usual regimen.

Presence of complications of diabetes

In patients who have been under regular review this knowledge will be available, but the development of a major complication provides an opportunity to undertake a more detailed assessment.

Retinopathy

Visual acuity should be tested and the optic fundi examined. Visual impairment may seriously reduce the patient's ability to look after the foot adequately. More detail can be obtained by fluorescein angiography. This may demonstrate areas of ischaemia which cannot be detected by other methods.

Renal function

Qualitative and quantitative measurement of the degree of proteinuria should be carried out. Blood urea and creatinine estimation give more detailed information about the degree of impairment of renal function. Renal failure is one of the important causes of death in these patients and once proteinuria occurs there is usually a progressive deterioration in renal function. Infection, ischaemia and papillary necrosis are important lesions which may aggravate the renal failure.

Cardiac disease

The history will give details of past episodes of angina pectoris, myocardial infarction or cardiac failure. An electrocardiogram may give evidence of ischaemia or a conduction defect which is not detected by physical examination. This information is important in determining the fitness of the patient for any operation that may be contemplated. In some patients, when major vascular surgery is planned, it is necessary to perform coronary angiography or isotope scanning of the heart. This part of the assessment is important because myocardial infarction is the commonest cause of postoperative death in these patients.

Social factors

The care that can be given depends to a large extent on the socioeconomic circumstances. The problems encountered in caring for patients in an affluent Western society are different from those in less wealthy communities. At an individual level, the patient's home circumstances are important. Successful outpatient treatment and prevention of recurrent lesions depends very much on the ability of the patient to cooperate in the treatment plan. The availability of domiciliary nursing services and the health of the patient's spouse can have a great influence on the outcome. There is a group of patients with neuropathy, usually men aged 50–70, often with a high alcohol intake, who have little insight into the potential seriousness of their condition and who are unable to achieve the standard of personal care necessary for control of the condition. Morbidity and mortality are high in this group.

LOCAL ASSESSMENT

Local assessment is directed at determining the severity of infection, arterial disease and neuropathy. The presence and severity of infection determines the urgency with which treatment must be undertaken. Once this has been established, the major part of the assessment is to decide the relative severity of arterial disease and neuropathy. It is important to remember that the severity of the arterial disease is the major determinant of healing.

Infection

Infection, which may vary in severity from a small area of redness around a bunion to a life-threatening spreading anaerobic cellulitis is the dominant feature in patients presenting acutely (see Ch. 8). Early diagnosis and control of infection is very important in the management of these patients. Invasive infection must be treated vigorously to prevent spread which will inevitably lead to further loss of tissue. Redness of the skin may result from friction or developing ischaemic necrosis. If the skin is intact, attention should be directed to relieving the source of injury. If the skin is broken and there is surrounding inflammation, it is usually wise to assume that there is infection and treat with antibiotics.

Samples of any exudate or pus from the lesion should be sent to the laboratory for microscopic examination and culture. It is important that the specimen be sent in transport medium to preserve anaerobic organisms, particularly if there is likely to be any delay in starting cultures. Any open wound or ulcer will be contaminated with bacteria and will present a portal through which infection may become established, although invasive infection will not necessarily occur. Healthy granulation tissue provides an excellent barrier to the spread of infection although contaminating organisms will usually be found. It is important to distinguish between contaminated and infected wounds, because the former require careful observation but the latter require aggressive chemotherapy.

The immediately dangerous infections are spreading anaerobic sepsis, which is a serious threat to life, and the presence of a deep abscess, which causes progressive tissue damage. The features of these infections have been described on page 123.

The presence of general features of infection depend on the amount of tissue involved and the presence of pus. High fever and marked leucocytosis indicate an abscess, usually deep in the foot. An increased tendency to hyperglycaemia and ketosis is also indirect evidence of uncontrolled infection.

Radiology of the foot

Radiographs of the foot should be taken if there is any suspicion of deep infection, e.g. abscess or osteomyelitis. The signs which suggest the presence of osteomyelitis are:

1. Bone destruction. In these patients this is commonly seen at a metatarsophalangeal joint or in the interphalangeal joint of the great toe (Fig. 9.1). In the earlier cases these will be small erosions at the margins of the bone; later there is obvious destruction of the articular surfaces (Fig. 9.2).
2. Sequestrum formation and subperiosteal new bone may be seen but are uncommon in these patients.
3. Gas in the tissues. A small amount of gas may be seen along the track between an ulcer and an underlying joint. Gas may also be seen in an abscess cavity in the foot. Large amounts of subcutaneous gas, especially if it extends towards the leg, may indicate a serious anaerobic infection.
4. Soft tissue swelling may often be seen due to the oedema which accompanies inflammation.

The changes of bone destruction described above may appear identical to the changes which accompany neuropathic degeneration in the metatarsophalangeal joint region (see p. 123). If there is clinical evidence of infection in the foot, evidence of bone destruction should be assumed to be due to infection. The same conclusion should be reached if a communication between a joint and an ulcer can be demonstrated by gentle probing or if tendon is visible in the base of an ulcer. Radiological signs of neuropathic

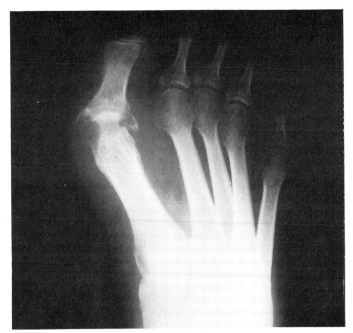

Fig. 9.1 Early signs of infection. Erosions around margins of head of metatarsal. Patient had recurrent episodes of 'cellulitis'. Radiograph was normal 6 weeks previously.

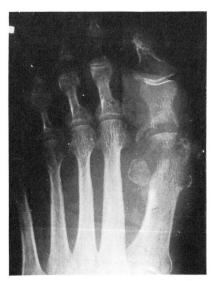

Fig. 9.2 Later signs of infection. Obvious evidence of destruction of metatarsophalangeal joint.

degeneration between the tarsal joints are unlikely to influence the outcome of infection or ulcer in the forefoot.

There are several radiological signs of accompanying arterial disease. In severe ischaemia there may be a generalized osteoporosis in the bones of the foot. In addition, calcification of the metatarsal or digital vessels is commonly seen (Figs. 9.3, 9.4). It is not necessary to take special soft tissue radiographs to search for this because these changes, although they reflect prolonged hyperglycaemia, do not indicate the presence of arterial disease which will impair healing of foot lesions.

Arterial disease

Presence of pain

If the nerve supply to the foot is intact, ulcers and gangrene are painful. The absence of pain means that neuropathy is present but gives no indication of the severity of the arterial disease. On the other hand, ischaemic rest pain means that there is major artery obstruction. The features of this pain are quite characteristic. It occurs at rest (in contrast to ischaemic exercise pain or intermittent claudication which, by definition, occurs only on exercise). In its mildest forms the patient may complain only of coldness and numbness of the toes at night and this symptom may be difficult to distinguish from the symptoms of peripheral neuropathy. In more severe cases the patient has a constant nagging, severe pain in the toes and foot.

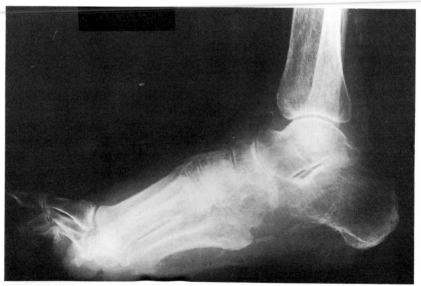

Fig. 9.3 Calcification of arteries. Extensive calfication of the posterior tibial artery and its terminal branches. Same patient as Fig. 3.7.

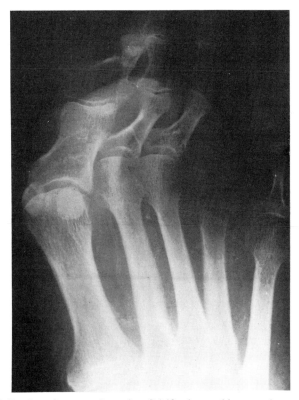

Fig. 9.4 Calcification of metatarsal arteries. Calcification to this extent is commonly seen in the feet of diabetics.

The pain is worse when the patient is recumbent and may be eased by hanging the leg over the side of the bed or walking on the cold floor. The patient may only be able to sleep by sitting in a chair with the legs dependent. This last feature distinguishes ischaemic pain from pain associated with infection because pain due to infection is relieved by elevation of the limb.

Palpation of pulses

If the ankle pulses are palpable there is enough blood reaching the foot to allow a local amputation to heal. In general, the need for a below-the-knee or higher amputation in such a patient represents a therapeutic disaster, although it is recognized that, in a few cases, so much tissue damage has occurred before presentation that it is impossible to save the foot. The presence of one or other of the dorsalis pedis and posterior tibial pulses means that either the axial arterial system is patent, or the collateral vessels are very well developed.

If the pulses are impalpable, there is either arterial obstruction or so much oedema of the foot that normal arteries are impalpable. The pulses higher in the leg should be examined. If the popliteal pulse is absent but the femoral pulse is present, the superficial femoral artery is obstructed. However, this does not necessarily mean that arterial obstruction is the cause of the lesion or that local amputation will fail. There may be sufficient collateral circulation to maintain the viability of the foot and even to allow local healing to occur, although the time taken for wounds to heal may be prolonged. If the popliteal pulse is present then the femoral artery is patent, although it may be stenosed. In these circumstances, if major arteries are obstructed, the site of occlusion must be distal to the popliteal arteries. The presence of a popliteal pulse and the absence of both ankle pulses is rare in non-diabetic subjects because obstruction to the vessels below the knee is uncommon in the absence of diabetes. Thus, although inexperienced observers often find the popliteal pulse difficult to feel, it is a sign of great importance in these patients. If the femoral pulse is absent, more distal pulses are unlikely to be present. This situation, which indicates the presence of obstruction to the iliac arteries, is relatively uncommon in diabetics. Figure 9.5 provides a summary of these findings.

Temperature of the skin

Feeling the temperature of the skin may be a good guide to the adequacy of the circulation to the limb — coldness is an important sign of ischaemia. In patients with femoral artery obstruction there is often a distinct change

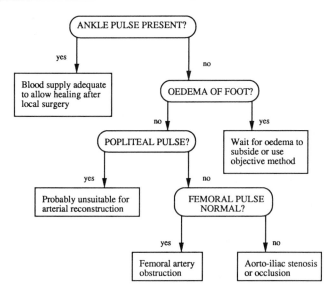

Fig. 9.5 Flow chart for findings on palpation of pulses.

in temperature of the skin at the level of the midpoint of the tibia. In addition, the skin over the knee on the affected side may be warmer because of the presence of subcutaneous collateral vessels. A cold foot with a temperature gradient at midtibia suggests a femoral artery obstruction producing moderate to severe ischaemia. If there is obstruction above the origin of the profunda femoris artery the temperature gradient may be at mid thigh level. Classification of patients according to the temperature of the skin of the foot can provide a useful basis for determining the likely success of local amputation (Williams et al 1974).

The importance of areas of increased redness or warmth in indicating areas which are inflamed as the result of repetitive mechanical trauma has been mentioned on page 88.

Neuropathy

A detailed clinical examination of the central and peripheral nervous system should be undertaken. The possible findings can be inferred from the discussion in Chapter 4. They include changes in pupillary reactions, cranial nerve lesions, evidence of neuropathy involving the upper limbs especially mononeuropathies and evidence of proximal muscle wasting associated with the syndrome of amyotrophy.

 Examination of the foot and leg reveals most of the signs. Inspection of the posture of the foot is very important. Clawing of the toes, especially if accompanied by thinning of the plantar fat pad so that the metatarsal heads are more prominent, suggests that there is neuropathy affecting the small muscles of the foot. Local areas of hyperkeratosis may be followed by painless plantar ulcers which are a characteristic result of diabetic neuropathy. Ulcers may be present at other sites of pressure, e.g. the interphalangeal joint of the great toe, the base of the fifth metatarsal and the dorsum of interphalangeal joints of clawed toes. The absence of dark necrotic tissue is typical. The deformity produced by neuropathic joints is usually seen in the region of the intertarsal joints. This may result in a deformity which is so disabling that the patient may not be able to wear ordinary shoes. Neuropathic change involving the metatarsal bones will be detected on X-ray (page 123).

Sensory testing, particularly for light touch and pin prick, should be performed. In the presence of a plantar ulcer there will be decreased perception of pain in the toes and forefoot. Loss of vibration sense at the ankle is very common. This sense is also lost in some non-diabetic elderly patients and does not on its own indicate diabetic neuropathy. However, loss of vibration sense at the knee or higher levels is definitely abnormal.

Changes in tendon reflexes occur in parallel with the severity of the neuropathy. Loss of the ankle reflex accompanies loss of vibration sense at the ankle as part of the ageing process and these signs are not of major significance. Loss of the patellar tendon reflex indicates moderately severe neuropathy.

The function of the small muscles of the foot is difficult to test clinically, although it can be inferred from the postural changes described above and can be easily demonstrated by electrophysiological testing. Weakness of the movements of the ankle and toes, which indicates a more severe neuropathy, can be demonstrated in about half the patients with lesions. Occasionally the patient will have foot drop from a mononeuropathy involving the common peroneal nerve.

Autonomic neuropathy may be detected at the bedside by observing the fall in blood pressure which occurs when the subject stands up from a lying position. The more detailed tests of autonomic function have been described in Chapter 4.

At the end of the examination an assessment must be made of the relative severity of infection, ischaemia and neuropathy. This can often be done adequately by the standard clinical examination outlined above, but on many occasions there remain doubts, particularly about the adequacy of the blood supply. The tests which may be used to provide more information are the subject of the next section.

SPECIAL TESTS

The assessment discussed above uses standard clinical methods; this section discusses additional investigations which may be performed. Some of these tests, e.g. Doppler ultrasound, radionuclide scanning and angiography are available in most general hospitals. Others, although often simple in concept, are used only in centres with special interests or where research projects are being undertaken.

Special tests are available for studying the functions of both the autonomic and somatic parts of the nervous system. The changes in nerve conduction have been described on page 47 and the tests which may be used to test autonomic function are given on page 55. The tests for somatic neuropathy do not provide any information which might be useful in establishing the short-term prognosis although the persistence of neuropathy may, of course, be an important factor in determining the development of subsequent lesions.

Assessment of the blood supply of the foot

This topic is addressed in detail for several reasons. First, there has been much new information in recent years so our understanding of these problems has improved. Second, the information regarding the use of these tests is distributed widely in the literature and its collection might serve as a useful reference source.

Measurement of arterial blood pressure

An occlusion in an artery will result in a fall in blood pressure in the arterial bed distal to the occlusion. Maintenance of the circulation to the distal tissues depends on collateral pathways. If these are good, e.g. around the elbow, an arterial occlusion will have only minor effects. If there are no available alternative channels, e.g. in the retina, serious consequences will follow. The clinical signs distal to an arterial obstruction include loss of arterial pulsation and reduced distal blood pressure.

The ability to measure arterial blood pressure in the legs has had a major impact on the practice of vascular surgery and one of these tests is an essential routine part of the assessment of patients. Several techniques will be discussed. They all rely on detection of returning blood flow distal to a cuff in which the pressure is deflated from suprasystolic levels, and are identical in principle to the palpatory method for measuring brachial artery pressure. These techniques are of considerable benefit because they allow the measurement of blood pressure with acceptable accuracy, over the whole range, from normal to less than 20 mm mercury. This allows a quantitative assessment of the severity of the arterial disease to be made because the level of the systolic pressure measured at the ankle relates well to the clinical state of the patient (Yao 1970). The sensitivity of the assessment can be increased if the pressure is measured before and after exercise or some other hyperaemic stimulus. If there is significant arterial stenosis, a fall in pressure at the ankle will occur after exercise and this is the basis of a widely used screening test for patients with vascular disease.

Before these tests were available the assessment of the patient by physical examination depended largely on the ability to feel the ankle pulses (see page 136). This sign is very susceptible to variation between observers and the pulses may be masked by the presence of oedema. In addition, although the pulses are absent, the leg may be symptomless.

Doppler ultrasound. If a continuous beam of sound is transmitted through tissues it will be reflected from various objects in its path. If these objects are moving, e.g. blood cells, the frequency of the reflected wave will be altered and this change will be proportional to the velocity of movement (Fig 9.6). This is the basis of the Doppler ultrasound method.

The apparatus consists of a probe, which contains both transmitting and receiving elements, connected to a box which generates the ultrasound and processes the returning waves. These are manipulated electronically to produce a signal which may be fed either to a speaker to produce an audible output or a chart recorder to produce a visible tracing. The main use of this apparatus is to act as a very sensitive pulse detector. It can be used over arteries as large as the femoral arteries and as small as the digital arteries in the fingers.

The method is most valuable in measuring pressure in the arteries low in the leg. The occluding cuff is applied to the lower part of the calf, and the

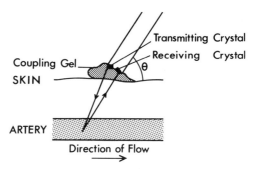

Fig. 9.6   Doppler principle. The frequency shift of the returning sound depends on the transmitted frequency, the angle between the beam and the moving particles and the velocity of the particles.

probe is placed successively over the posterior tibial artery behind the medial malleolus and the dorsalis pedis artery over the metatarsal bones. If the dorsalis pedis artery is absent, a signal from the terminal branch of the peroneal artery can usually be heard more laterally on the dorsum of the foot, anterior to the medial border of the fibula. The systolic pressure should be recorded from both the posterior tibial and dorsalis pedis arteries.

In normal subjects, the ankle pressure is equal to or slightly higher than the brachial artery pressure, but in diabetics occlusion of one of the calf arteries might produce marked differences in the measured pressures. Pressure may be expressed in absolute terms or, more commonly, as the ratio of ankle/brachial pressure, sometimes called the Pressure Index (PI). In normal subjects this is greater than 0.9.

Placing appropriate cuffs at other appropriate levels in the leg may allow estimates of the pressure in the vessels of the upper part of the calf and the thigh. These estimates bear a less certain relationship to intravascular pressure than measurements made at the ankle and their use in this way is not recommended.

The PI is a valuable guide to the severity of the ischaemia and to prognosis. However, there is one serious qualification which must be remembered with diabetic patients. If the artery wall is calcified it may not be compressed when the occlusion cuff is inflated. This means that a distal flow signal will still be audible although the cuff pressure is well above systolic pressure. In these circumstances the ankle pressure measurement is of no value. An experienced observer will be alerted when hearing an abnormal flow signal in an artery in which the pressure is measured at or near normal levels. There is little data on the frequency with which this occurs. It is difficult to predict if an artery will be compressible even if calcification is seen radiologically. Carter (1973) found that in four out of five limbs with extensive calcification, the indirectly measured pressure was over 10 mm Hg higher than the pressure measured directly. Gibbons et al (1979), found indirectly measured pressures of more than 200 mm Hg in 22 of 150 patients in their report. We have demonstrated (Quigley et al 1990a) that, when compared with skin perfusion pressure (see p. 142), ankle blood pressure is raised in diabetic subjects over the whole range of pressures, even when those with incompressible arteries are excluded.

Mercury strain gauge.   This method has been described by Nielsen et al (1973). The pulse detector consists of a thin silastic tube filled with mercury which makes contact with copper wires at each end of the column. This gauge is placed around a digit or limb. With each heart beat there is a small pulse in the tissues and this causes elongation of the gauge. With the change in length, there is a proportional change in the electrical resistance of the column of mercury and this can be detected using a Wheatstone bridge or other appropriate circuit. The output can be led to a chart recorder. Blood pressure can be measured in two ways. Using an AC circuit the cuff pressure at which the pulsation returns can be recorded as the systolic pressure. Alternatively, using a DC circuit, systolic pressure can be recorded as the cuff pressure at which the volume of the part begins to increase (Fig. 9.7). The pressures measured using the two techniques are closely related to each other and to the pressure obtained with the Doppler ultrasound method. The equipment is available as a package (e.g. Plethysmograph SP2, Medimatic, Copenhagen, Denmark) or the components (e.g. Parks Plethysmograph, Beaverton, Oregon, USA) can be attached to a recorder of the user's choice.

A cuff placed above the ankle allows the measurement of the systolic blood pressure at that level and the interpretation of this information has been discussed. If a cuff is placed around the base of a toe with a strain gauge distal to it, pressure can also be measured in the toe.

Pulse volume recorder.   This represents a modern version of the oscillometer which was one of the earliest instruments used in the assessment of patients with vascular disease. In its present form it consists of a series of sphygmomanometer cuffs which are placed around the leg at several levels. The cuffs are inflated to subdiastolic levels and the pressure changes transmitted to them from the underlying arteries can be recorded. The

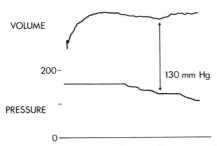

Fig. 9.7   Measurement of toe blood pressure. The systolic pressure is indicated by the point where the baseline shifts as the volume of the digit increases when blood returns to the digit.

equipment is available as a package and is widely used in vascular laboratories in the USA (Raines et al 1976). It is used to make qualitative assessments of arterial pulsations and as a pulse detector for measurement of segmental blood pressure.

The idea of using the blood pressure measured at several levels in the limb to map the distribution of the arterial disease is an attractive one. With this equipment, cuffs may be placed high on the thigh, above and below the knee and above the ankle, and an estimate of arterial pressure made at each level. A pressure gradient between adjacent levels or between corresponding sites on opposite limbs may indicate arterial narrowing or occlusion in the segment above the lower cuff. But the method is of limited use. The estimate of thigh blood pressure is falsely high because of the narrowness of the cuff in relation to the circumference of the thigh. The problems of calcified arteries, as mentioned above, may also exist.

In diabetics, this technique has been used in association with Doppler measurements to predict healing of ulcers and the results of forefoot amputation but the accuracy of this prediction is not high (Gibbons et al 1979). The method is satisfactory for the measurement of ankle blood pressure and it has been found empirically to be useful for other purposes.

Measurement of blood pressure in the skin

The measurement of ankle blood pressure, which is the simplest of the methods to use, does not provide adequate information for assessing prognosis in many patients (Gibbons et al 1979, Sumner 1983). Assessment of more distal blood supply is needed. One method for this, the measurement of toe blood pressure, has been described above. There are several methods for estimating blood pressure in the skin. They use external counter-pressure and vary according to how the blood flow in the skin is detected.

Isotope clearance.   This method was originally described by Lassen & Holstein (1974), who studied the clearance of ^{133}Xe from the skin (Fig. 9.8). More recently [^{99m}Tc] pertechnetate has been shown to give comparable results. In this technique a small volume (0.05 ml) of radioisotope is mixed with a vasodilator (histamine or sodium nitroprusside) to give maximum local vasodilatation and is injected into the skin. The rate of clearance of the isotope is monitored via the ratemeter and recording system. External pressure is applied over the injection site, using a sphygmomanometer cuff. The end point is reached when the pressure in the cuff is high enough to just prevent further clearance of isotope from the skin. This is called the skin perfusion pressure (SPP). In normal subjects the pressure recorded is between the diastolic and mean blood pressure and it is presumed that in ischaemic areas, where pulsatile flow is much reduced, that the SPP reflects the local arterial perfusion pressure.

Photoelectric plethysmography.   In this method a light-emitting diode

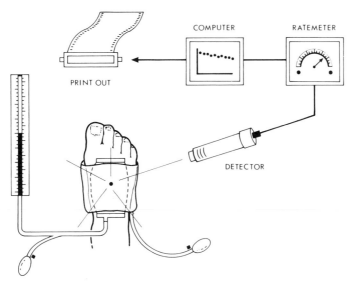

Fig. 9.8 Measurement of skin blood pressure. Pressure is applied over the depot of radioisotope by a sphygmomanometer cuff. The rate meter is connected to a computer to facilitate calculations.

is placed on the skin and transmits light into the tissues. The amount of reflected light detected by a photocell is proportional to the amount of haemoglobin in the tissues. As with the mercury strain gauge, the apparatus can be used in either AC or DC mode. External pressure is used to blanch the skin and, as the pressure is reduced, the pressure at which a flow signal returns is the skin perfusion pressure. This gives values similar to those obtained using the isotope clearance method (Holstein et al 1979b). Using this method Holstein and Lassen (1980) found that a foot lesion was certain to heal if the pressure in the skin was recorded as 30 mm Hg or higher. Lee et al (1979) used similar apparatus to study the cutaneous circulation around bed sores and leg ulcers.

Laser Doppler flowmetry.   A laser source is applied to the skin and the returning reflected light analysed for changes in wavelength. These changes are produced, according to the Doppler effect, by moving red blood cells in the superficial layer of the skin. The skin blood pressure can be estimated by a method similar to that used with photoelectric plethysmography.

Isotope perfusion scanning.   These methods involve systemic administration of radioactive material and subsequent examination of the leg with a gamma camera, to determine the amount of radioisotope present and/or its distribution. The rate of accumulation of ^{99m}Tc in the foot following intra-arterial injection has been used to estimate the blood flow velocity in the limb. Shionoya et al (1981) have demonstrated that the movement of isotope is slower in more ischaemic limbs and that this is reversible with surgery. The pattern of accummulation of radioisotope has been used for several purposes.

1. Prediction of ulcer healing. If the local blood supply is adequate to allow healing of an ulcer, there will be hyperaemia in the surrounding skin and a larger proportion of the injected isotope will accumulate in this area. This increased radioactivity can be measured. The most commonly used measurement is the ratio of radioactivity in the surrounding skin to the radioactivity in the ulcer. A ratio has been used to try to minimize the importance of changes in skin blood flow which might result from such variables as anxiety, temperature changes and smoking. The critical value of the ratio varies in different reports from 2.3 to 3.5 (Siegel et al 1975, Johnson & Patten 1977). These authors suggest that the indications for using this method include delayed healing despite the presence of ankle pulses, and absent ankle pulse but an ankle pressure (using the Doppler technique), of more than 55 mm Hg. Patients with pressures lower than 50 mm Hg may be considered for reconstructive vascular surgery (see previous section).

2. ^{99m}Tc-phosphate imaging following intravenous injection has been used to provide evidence about the blood supply and the presence of osteomyelitis (Lawrence et al 1983). Isotope scanning is more sensitive than radiographs in detecting osteomyelitis of the small bones of the foot (Park et al 1982).

3. The patterns of distribution of ^{201}Th injected intravenously is analogous to the distribution observed in the myocardium in patients with ischaemic heart disease. A moderately ischaemic area may not show perfusion initially but the isotope will gradually accumulate and be visible on a delayed scan. An initial 'hot spot' indicates a good blood supply (Ohta 1985). The factors which determine the distribution of isotope to the tissues of the leg are poorly understood. It is important that the technique of injection should ensure adequate mixing of the isotope with the blood. It is clear that certain patterns of distribution can be recognized (Rhodes et al 1976). In one, the isotope is distributed roughly in proportion to the muscle mass. If symptoms of ischaemia are present, this pattern is said to represent large vessel disease. In another pattern, the isotope has a more patchy distribution and this is said to represent the presence of small vessel disease, presumably involving arterioles and capillaries. These different patterns are easily demonstrated but their interpretation is open to question particularly as there is no clear explanation as to why the isotope should distribute preferentially to the skin if there is small vessel disease present. There is no histological evidence to support the interpretation given.

These isotope perfusion tests are easily applied in any centre with a nuclear medicine department but their usefulness in aiding the management of large numbers of patients has not been established.

Measurement of transcutaneous oxygen tension TcpO2 In this method (Matsen et al 1980), the partial pressure of the oxygen which diffuses to the surface of the skin is measured by an electrode heated to 43–44°C. Under these circumstances the measured $TcpO_2$ reflects the pO_2 in the underlying arteries because the blood in the capillaries becomes arterialized as a consequence of the vasodilatation produced by the heating. In patients with arterial disease the systemic pO_2 may be normal but the $TcpO_2$ in the limb reduced because of the decreased delivery of oxygenated blood to the skin. This method has been used to classify the severity of the arterial disease and predict amputation healing (Clyne et al 1982, Katsamouris et al 1984). The results have been expressed as the absolute value of the $TcpO_2$ or as the ratio between the level of $TcpO_2$ in the leg to the $TcpO_2$ in some area with a normal arterial supply, e.g. the chest wall or upper arm.

We have studied the value of $TcpO_2$ measurement in comparison with the radioisotope measurement of SPP and SVR (see p. 149). Our results suggest that the absolute value of $TcpO_2$ is the preferred criterion for expressing the results. Our hypothesis, that $TcpO_2$ is affected by both the SPP, reflecting large artery disease, and the SVR, reflecting microvascular disease, has been supported by the evidence (Quigley et al 1990b). This suggests that the presence of microvascular disease whether due to diabetes, hypertension or other cause should be considered when interpreting $TcpO_2$ readings.

Imaging of arteries

The tests described above provide valuable information about the effects of any arterial disease which is present and their widespread application has made a major contribution to the care of these patients. Information regarding the anatomy of the arterial occlusions is essential before reconstructive arterial surgery is undertaken. The patterns of disease seen are described in Chapter 3 and the types of arterial surgery performed are discussed in Chapter 10. Images of the arteries can be obtained in several ways.

Intra-arterial injection of contrast (arteriography). This is the standard method. A needle or catheter is inserted into the arterial tree proximal to the arterial occlusions and contrast injected. This procedure is moderately unpleasant for the patient and there is a small, but definite, risk of arterial injury as a consequence of the procedure. The sorts of images produced are shown in Fig. 3.4.

Intravenous injection of contrast (digital subtraction angiography). This method has become available in the past 10 years. It uses the power of a (digital) computer to enhance the radiographic image so that views of the arteries can be obtained following intravenous injection. The method has the disadvantages that it is expensive, uses large volumes of contrast and the quality of the image is inadequate in 25–30% of cases. Image quality can be improved and the dose of contrast reduced by intra-arterial injection.

Duplex ultrasound. In recent years, machines have been available which combine the Doppler principle described above with B-mode ultrasound to produce both an image of the artery and information regarding the blood flow within it. The combination of the two modalities is called 'Duplex Scanning'. This method has been particularly useful in examining the carotid bifurcation but developments in the apparatus have been made which allow the method to be applied to many areas in the arterial system. It is likely that these improvements will result in the equipment being used more widely and replacing angiography in some situations.

The indications for arteriography are the same in diabetics and non-diabetics. If it is considered that the foot is unlikely to survive without arterial reconstruction, if the patient is fit for operation and if the foot is not irreversibly damaged by ischaemia or infection, arteriography should be performed to determine if reconstruction is feasible. This decision can be made on clinical grounds in a patient with a history of rest pain or disabling intermittent claudication or with ischaemic ulcers of gangrene. It is not necessary to perform angiography in patients in whom the ankle pulses are palpable or the SPP is greater than 50 mm Hg or the ankle PI greater than 0.5 (provided the arteries are not calcified). The information required from the arteriogram must include the state of the arteries above and below the occlusion. This usually means that the radiologist must display the arterial tree from the level of the aorta to the ankle.

APPLICATIONS

An adequate blood supply is essential for healing of ulcers and gangrene of the leg or foot regardless of the role of infection or neuropathy in the development of the lesion. Thus an accurate assessment of the blood supply is necessary for the planning of optimal treatment. If the blood supply is wrongly judged to be adequate, attempts at local treatment of the lesions will not result in healing. This often means that the patient undergoes multiple local procedures, spends a large amount of time in hospital and becomes increasingly demoralized and frail and still often requires a major amputation. However, even if arterial occlusion is present, the blood supply to the foot may be good enough to allow healing. In these circumstances it is wrong to submit the patient to the hazards of arterial surgery.

The two questions asked most commonly are:
1. Will an ulcer or local gangrene heal?
2. Will an amputation performed at a particular level heal?

The methods described above give answers of greater precision than has hitherto been possible although it should not be thought that the predictions are invariably correct.

Measurement of ankle pressure

Carter (1973) suggested that healing of the foot was unlikely if the ankle systolic pressure was less than 55 mm Hg. Above this level, the lesion would heal in almost all non-diabetics but amputation was necessary in 14 of 66 diabetics with pressures over 55 mm Hg. Raines et al (1976) found empirically that healing was unlikely if the ankle pressure was less than 55 mm Hg in non-diabetic and less than 80 mm Hg in diabetic patients. It is said that on average the ankle pressure is higher in diabetics than in non-diabetics with lesions but this probably reflects the role of neuropathy and infection in the diabetic subjects. Arterial calcification would also tend to produce higher pressure readings.

Similar controversy exists over the role of these measurements in predicting the healing of amputation wounds. A centre with a large experience of the surgery in these patients (Gibbons et al 1979) found that for foot amputations a low ankle pressure (less than 70 mm Hg) was as frequently in those whose amputations healed as in those in whom amputation failed. In the same report an ankle pressure of under 70 mm Hg occurred in 22 of 48 below-knee amputations (BKA) which healed successfully. Several reports have indicated that the level of the ankle systolic pressure is a useful predictor of healing of BKA . Barnes et al (1976) and Pollock & Ernst (1980) both reported that healing was likely if the ankle pressure was at least 70 mm mercury. However, healing will occur in some patients with lower ankle pressures so that using this criterion to exclude the possibility of a BKA will result in the performance of a larger number of higher amputations which are more disabling.

There are two major limitations to the application of ankle pressure measurements in diabetic patients. The first is the problem of arterial calcification and the second is the relatively poor predictive value of ankle pressure measurements for healing of lesions of the forefoot, which are very common in diabetics. A normal ankle systolic pressure and a normal pulse signal at the ankle are evidence of a blood supply adequate to allow elective foot surgery and to permit healing of lesions of the forefoot. Despite these limitations, the measurement of ankle pressure using the Doppler apparatus is the single most valuable adjunct to the assessment of the blood supply of the foot in these patients.

Measurement of blood pressure distally in the foot

It is reasonable to believe that assessment of the blood supply closer to the lesion would give more useful information than measurement of ankle blood pressure. The value of measurement of toe blood pressure has been well documented. It has several important applications:

Classification of patients. A toe systolic pressure over 20 mm Hg is found in more than 70% of patients with rest pain or ischaemic ulcers but in less than 20% of patients who present with intermittent claudication (Tonnesen et al 1980).

Development of ulcers in diabetics. Diabetic patients have a higher pressure gradient between toe and ankle than non-diabetics. The highest gradients, i.e. the lowest toe pressures, are found in patients with ulcers or gangrene of the foot (Faris 1975). This probably relates to the finding of proliferative intimal changes and occlusion of digital and metatarsal arteries.

Prediction of healing of ulcers or gangrene. If the toe pressure remains under 20 mm Hg, the chances of a foot lesion healing are less than 10%. If the toe pressure is over 30 mm Hg, healing can be confidently expected following local treatment (Holstein & Lassen 1980, Ramsey et al 1983) (Fig. 9.9). A rise in the pressure following arterial reconstruction permits local healing if the pressure rises above 30 mm Hg. These results provide a much clearer discrimination than has been obtained from other methods of segmental pressure measurement.

Toe blood pressure measurement is technically demanding and may be difficult when the pressure is low. The methods for measuring blood pressure in the skin are an alternative to the measurement of toe blood pressure and provide more valuable information than the ankle pressure. Measurement of skin perfusion pressure for the prediction of healing of major amputations has been reported by Holstein et al (1979a and c). If the skin perfusion pressure was over 30 mm Hg at the proposed site of the skin incision, major wound complications occurred in less than 10% of patients. However there was a very high frequency of wound complications and

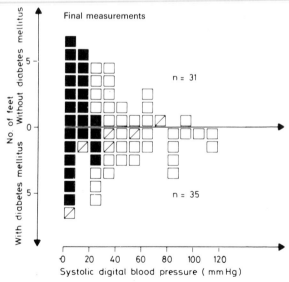

Fig. 9.9 Effect of toe systolic pressure on the healing of lesions of the foot. Closed squares – healing, square with diagonal line – healing following local amputation, open squares – major amputation. (From Holstein & Lassen, 1980).

failure of healing if the skin perfusion pressure was below this value. The method, as applied by Moore (1973), involved intradermal injection of ^{133}Xe dissolved in saline into the pretibial skin 10 cm below the tibial tuberosity. This level corresponds to the site of the anterior skin incision for a BKA (see p. 183 for technique of amputation) and is the site at which ischaemic necrosis most commonly occurs. The rate of disappearance of ^{133}Xe depends on capillary blood flow, and this can be calculated from measurements of the rate of decrease of the radioactivity. A critical level of flow of 2.6 ml/100 g/min predicted healing in those limbs with greater flow and failure of healing if the flow was less than the critical level. A subsequent report from this group (Malone et al 1979) indicated the results that could be obtained with careful assessment, good surgery and aggressive rehabilitation. In 133 patients (two thirds of whom were diabetic) there were no postoperative deaths, 89% of amputations healed and all unilateral BKA patients were fitted with prostheses.

Our own experience is predominantly with the radioisotope clearance method (p. 142). Analysis of our results showed that skin blood pressure (SPP) was a predictor of both local healing and the overall prognosis for the patient (Faris et al 1988).

Diagnosis of microangiopathy

The histological diagnosis of microangiopathy has been discussed earlier (p. 25). One of the major problems in determining the role of micro-vascular disease as a cause of foot lesions has been the lack of a test to diagnose microangiopathy in the living limb. We believe that data obtained from the radioisotope clearance test has largely overcome this deficiency.

When the various values for clearance and applied pressure (Fig. 9.10) are plotted (Fig. 9.11), a straight-line relationship is obtained. The slope of

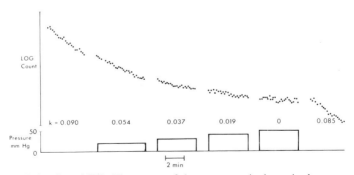

Fig. 9.10   Estimation of SPP. The output of the rate meter is shown in the upper part of the figure. The blocks in the lower part indicate the applied pressure which is increased in a stepwise fashion. The numbers indicate the clearance constant at each level of applied pressure.

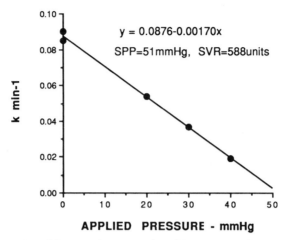

Fig. 9.11 Calculation of SPP and SVR. Data from Fig. 9.10. The SPP is the point where the plotted line meets the x axis. The SVR is the reciprocal of the slope (i.e. 1/0.0017).

this line has the dimensions flow/pressure which is equivalent to the reciprocal of resistance ($F = \Delta P/R$, $R = F/\Delta P$). The reciprocal of the slope is called the skin vascular resistance (SVR) and it has been our hypothesis that the level of skin resistance is an indicator of the presence of microangiopathy. We have produced several lines of evidence to support this view.

1. The SVR was increased in diabetic and hypertensive patients who developed ulcers and gangrene in the foot (Duncan & Faris 1986).

2. The SVR and SPP were independent predictors of healing of the foot in patients with ulcers or gangrene (Duncan & Faris 1986).

3. The SVR was raised in patients with Martorell's ulcers of the leg (Duncan & Faris 1985).

4. The SVR was raised in a group of diabetic patients with retinopathy compared with a matched group without retinopathy (Duncan & Faris 1991).

Independent confirmation has been obtained recently of the relationship between histological evidence of microangiopathy and SVR (Kastrup et al 1987).

The measurement of SPP provides evidence about the blood supply of the foot which is as valuable as that obtained by other methods, e.g. toe blood pressure. However, the SVR cannot be obtained by other methods and is an important independent predictor of outcome. This method has the additional advantage that it requires a cheap and easily available isotope in low dose and the counting equipment is inexpensive. Our prospective studies (Faris et al 1988) have shown that SVR is an independent predictor of healing of the foot. Thus we believe that microvascular disease is an important contributory factor in 20–30% of the patients we treat. Our study demonstrated that SPP, SVR and the age of the patient were the significant predictors of healing. (Note that, in this model, the ankle blood pressure was not a significant predictor.) Thus by using these three variables we can obtain an estimate of the probability of healing in any given patient (see Fig. 9.12). This test has enabled us to standardize the treatment of the diabetic patients we see, as shown in Figure 9.13. This has had two major advantages. First, patients with a low probability of healing are offered early amputation if arterial reconstruction is not feasible. This policy avoids futile local amputations and facilitates rehabilitation. Second, if the blood supply is adequate, arterial reconstruction is not needed even though arterial occlusion may be present. We believe we can avoid arterial bypass in some patients by using this information.

Some form of laboratory assessment is required in almost all patients presenting with a serious foot problem. The tests used vary with the interests and experience at various centres, but the following summary reflects our present views and is justified by the available evidence in the literature.

1. The use of the Doppler apparatus to demonstrate normal ankle pressures and waveforms is a reliable guide to the normality of the circulation.

2. If the Doppler studies are abnormal or if the patient has a lesion of the forefoot, some measure of forefoot perfusion is required. We prefer to measure SPP using the isotope clearance method but the other methods described are appropriate.

3. If the lesion is an ulcer of the leg, isotope perfusion studies may be used to assess the potential for healing.

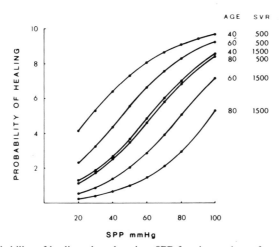

Fig. 9.12 Probability of healing plotted against SPP for given values of age and SVR.

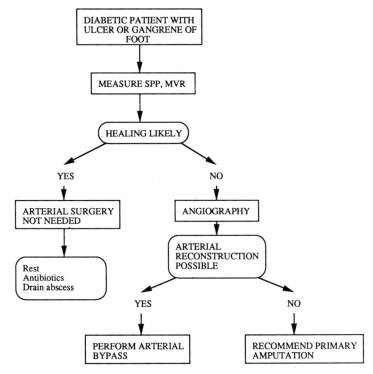

Fig. 9.13   Flow chart of plan of management based on estimates of SPP and SVR.

REFERENCES

Barnes R W, Shanik G D, Slaymaker E E 1976 An index of healing in below-knee
   amputation: leg blood pressure by Doppler ultrasound. Surgery 79: 13–20
Carter S A 1973 The relationship of distal systolic pressure to healing of skin lesions in
   limbs with arterial occlusive disease, with special reference to diabetes mellitus.
   Scandinavian Journal of Clinical & Laboratory Investigation Supplement 128,
   31: 239–243
Clyne C A C, Ryan J, Webster J H H, Chant A D B 1982 Oxygen tension on the skin of
   ischaemic legs. American Journal of Surgery 143: 315–318
Duncan H J, Faris I B 1985 Martorell's hypertensive ischemic leg ulcers are secondary to
   an increase in the local vascular resistance. Journal of Vascular Surgery 2: 581–584
Duncan H J, Faris I B 1986 Skin vascular resistance and skin perfusion pressure as
   predictors of healing of ischaemic lesion of the lower limb: influences of diabetes
   mellitus, hypertension and age. Surgery 99: 432–438
Duncan H J, Faris I B 1991 Microvascular resistance is raised in diabetic patients with
   microangiopathy. Diabetes Care (in press)
Faris I 1975 Small and large vessel disease in the development of foot lesions in diabetics.
   Diabetologia 11: 249–253
Faris I, Duncan H, Young C 1988 Factors affecting outcome of diabetic patients with foot
   ulcers or gangrene. Journal of Cardiovascular Surgery 29: 736–740
Gibbons G W, Wheelock F C Jr, Siembieda C, Hoar C S Jr, Rowbotham J L, Persson
   A B 1979 Non-invasive prediction of amputation level in diabetic patients. Archives of
   Surgery 114: 1253–1257

Holstein P, Dovey H, Lassen N A 1979a Wound healing in above-knee amputations in relation to skin perfusion pressure. Acta Orthopaedica Scandanavica 50: 59–66

Holstein P, Neilsen P E, Barras J-P 1979b Blood flow cessation at external pressure in the skin of normal human limbs. Photoelectric recordings compared to isotope washout and to local intra-arterial blood pressure. Microvascular Research 17: 71–79

Holstein P, Sager P, Lassen N A 1979c Wound healing in below-knee amputations in relation to skin perfusion pressure. Acta Orthopaedica Scandanavica 50: 49–58

Holstein P, Lassen N A 1980 Healing of ulcers of the feet correlated with distal blood pressure measurements in occlusive arterial disease. Acta Orthopaedica Scandanavica 51: 995–1006

Johnson W C, Patten D H 1977 Predictability of healing of ischaemic leg ulcers by radioisotopic and Doppler ultrasonic examination. American Journal of Surgery 133: 485–489

Kastrup J, Norgaard T, Parving H-H, Lassen N A 1987 Increased minimal vascular resistance and arteriolar hyalinosis in skin on the leg in insulin-dependent diabetic patients. Scandinavian Journal of Clinical and Laboratory Investigation 47: 475–482

Katsamouris A, Brewster D C, Megerman J, Cina C, Darling R C, Abbott W M 1984 Transcutaneous oxygen tension in selection of amputation level. American Journal of Surgery 147: 510–517

Lassen N A, Holstein P 1974 Use of radioisotopes in assessment of distal blood flow and distal blood pressure in arterial insufficiency. Surgical Clinics of North America 54: 39–55

Lawrence P F, Syverud J B, Disbro M A, Alazraki N 1983 Evaluation of Technetium-99m phosphate imaging for predicting skin ulcer healing. American Journal of Surgery 146: 746–750

Lee B Y, Trainor F S, Kavner D, Cresologo J A, Shaw W W, Madden J L 1979 Assessment of the healing potentials of ulcers of the skin by photoplethysmography. Surgery, Gynecology and Obstetrics 148: 232–239

Malone J M, Moore W S, Goldstone J, Malone S J 1979 Therapeutic and economic impact of a modern amputation programme. Annals of Surgery 189: 798–802

Matsen F A III, Whyss C R, Pedegana L R, Krugmire R B, Simmons C W, King R V, Burgess E M 1980 Transcutaneous oxygen tension measurements in peripheral vascular disease. Surgery Gynecology and Obstetrics 150: 525–528

Moore W S 1973 Determination of amputation level. Archives of Surgery 107: 798–802

Nielsen N A, Bell G, Lassen N A 1973 Strain gauge studies of distal blood pressure in normal subjects and in patients with peripheral arterial disease. Scandinavian Journal of Clinical Laboratory Investigation 31 (suppl 128): 103–109

Ohta T 1985 Non-invasive technique using Thallium-210 for predicting ischaemic ulcer healing of the foot. British Journal of Surgery 72: 892–895

Park H-M, Wheat J, Siddiqui A R, Burt R W, Robb J A, Ransburg R C, Kernek C B 1982 Scintigraphic evidence of diabetic osteomyelitis: concise communication. Journal of Nuclear Medicine 23: 569–573

Pollock S B Jr, Ernst C B 1980 Use of Doppler pressure measurements in predicting success in amputation of the leg. American Journal of Surgery 140: 103–106

Quigley F G, Faris I B, Duncan H J 1990a A comparison of Doppler ankle pressures and skin perfusion pressure in subjects with and without diabetes. Clinical Physiology (in press)

Quigley F, Faris I, Young C M A 1990b Factors affecting transcutaneous oxygen tension measurements in the assessment of the blood supply to the lower limb. (in press)

Raines J K, Darling R C, Buth J, Brewster D C, Austen W G 1976 Vascular laboratory criteria for the management of peripheral vascular disease of the lower extremities. Surgery 79: 21–29

Ramsey D E, Manke D A, Sumner D S 1983 Toe blood pressure, a valuable adjunct to ankle pressure measurement for assessing peripheral arterial disease. Journal of Cardiovascular Surgery 24: 43–48

Rhodes B A, Bader P, Stolz K, White R I, Siegel M E 1976. Assessment of peripheral vascular disease in patients with diabetes. Two case studies. Diabetes 25: 307–314.

Shionoya S, Hirai M, Kawai S, Ohta T, Seico T 1981 Hemodynamic study of ischaemic limb by velocity measurement in foot. Surgery 90: 10–19

Siegel M E, Giargiana F A, Rhodes B A, Williams G M, Wagner H N Jr 1975 Perfusion of ischemic ulcers of the extremity. Archives of Surgery 110: 265–168

Sumner D S 1983 Presidential address: noninvasive testing of vascular disease — fact, fancy, future. Surgery 93: 664–669

Tonnesen K H, Noer I, Paaske W, Sager P 1980 Classification of peripheral occlusive arterial disease based on symptoms, signs and distal blood pressure measurement. Acta Chirurgical Scandanavica 146: 101–104

Williams H T, Hutchinson K J, Brown G D 1974 Gangrene of the feet in diabetics. Archives of Surgery 108: 609–611

Yao S T 1970 Haemodynamic studies in peripheral arterial disease. British Journal of Surgery 57: 761–766

10. Management

This chapter describes the management of patients with infections, ulcers and gangrene. Their severity ranges from a minor area of skin loss resulting from wearing a new pair of shoes, to large areas of necrosis and spreading infection. The common factor is a break in the integrity of the skin. Once this occurs the most important barrier to infection has been lost and thus the risks to the patient are greatly increased. It cannot be emphasized often enough that the best management of these lesions is to prevent them from developing. In Chapter 7 the routine care that should be given to all diabetics was described and the treatment of early lesions was discussed. In this chapter detailed plans of management for more serious lesions will be given.

The indications for surgery will be discussed and the possible methods of treatment outlined. These include:

1. Conservative treatment
2. Drainage of an abscess
3. Minor amputation
4. Arterial reconstruction
5. Correction of deformity
6. Major amputation.

The techniques for performing the various operations are described later in the chapter.

INDICATIONS FOR OPERATION

Figure 10.1 shows a flow chart which may assist in determining the need for surgery in patients presenting with major foot problems. It is suggested that the questions to be asked in sequence are:

1. Is there an abscess or deep infection?
2. Is there ischaemic rest pain?
3. Is there joint or bone involvement?

If the answer to all these questions is 'no', non-operative treatment can be continued. The reasons for failure of conservative treatment are the

155

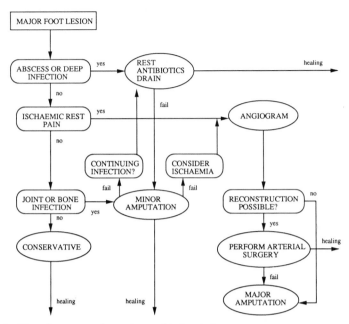

Fig. 10.1 Plan of treatment for patients with foot lesions.

presence of an abscess, joint or bone involvement, ischaemia, and failure to alleviate mechanical causes. It is essential at all stages to consider the possibility of an abscess in the foot. If this has been excluded, the next step is commonly to perform a local amputation in an attempt to secure healing. Failure of a local amputation is likely to be due to either infection or ischaemia. The former requires further local surgery, but the latter needs a successful arterial reconstruction if the foot is to be saved.

The two major indications for surgery in these patients are infection and ischaemia. Surgery is sometimes undertaken to correct deformity.

Infection

Abscess or deep infection

The clinical features have already been discussed. Minor infections which are presumed to be superficial should be treated by:

1. Rest
2. Culture exudate from wound
3. Antibiotics
4. Simple dressings, e.g. gauze soaked in saline or other non-irritant substance and changed daily
5. Later, modification of footwear to avoid repeated trauma.

If there is no improvement within 24–48 hours the patient should be admitted to hospital. Early admission may be required if there is significant ischaemia or if the patient cannot be cared for adequately at home.

Patients with severe infections should be admitted to hospital immediately. A suggested plan of management for these subjects is shown in Fig. 10.2. Great care should be taken not to overlook an abscess, because it cannot be cured by antibiotic therapy alone and local spread will result in continuing loss of tissue. For this reason early drainage of an abscess of the foot is important. The diagnosis of an abscess deep in the foot may be difficult but satisfactory healing will not occur unless deep infections are detected and drained. If there is tendon exposed in the base of an ulcer or if there is radiological evidence of osteomyelitis, the presence of a deep infection can safely be assumed.

The extent of the procedure that will be required is often underestimated. All necrotic tissue must be excised and all abscesses drained adequately. This must be carried out regardless of the presence of ischaemia and must be thorough and patient. Viable areas, including skin flaps, should be preserved and particular attention should be given to preserving weight-bearing skin. However skin will die if it has dead fat under it, so excision of dead tissue must take priority. Details of postoperative care are given on page 167.

During the 24–48 hours before the operation, the control of the diabetes can be improved, and antibiotic therapy (p. 73) will reduce the cellulitis and decrease the chance of the infection spreading after surgery.

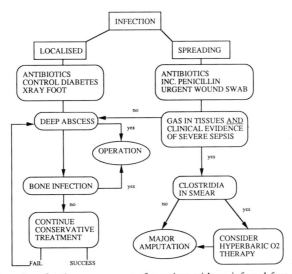

Fig. 10.2 Flow chart for the management of a patient with an infected foot.

Bone or joint infection

Infection which has involved a bone or joint is unlikely to resolve without excision of the affected area. The diagnosis can be made either by gentle probing of a sinus or by demonstrating exudation when a joint is moved. The radiological signs of infection (p. 121) may be difficult to distinguish from neuropathic joint change (see p. 123), but if there is an ulcer over a joint which shows these changes, it is likely that the joint is infected. These patients do not always undergo operation. In a foot with a normal blood supply, a more conservative approach using plaster of Paris immobilization (p. 108) may be advocated and, certainly in patients with leprosy, can be used successfully. However, it is more conventional in diabetic patients to excise the affected area, often using a ray amputation.

Severe anaerobic infection

This is the most serious outcome of infection in a foot and fortunately is a rare event. These patients have extending muscle necrosis that progresses rapidly up the leg. There may be swelling and tenderness in the calf and it will be apparent that the patient is seriously ill with fever, tachycardia and leucocytosis, and often septic shock. The commonest setting is in a patient who has undergone a partial foot amputation. In these circumstances, after restoration of the circulating blood volume and administration of large doses of antibiotics, a major amputation must be undertaken urgently. The possible use of hyperbaric oxygen therapy has been discussed on page 72.

Failure to drain adequately or excise infected tissue is a very common cause of failure of local treatment. The surgeon is often faced with the difficult decision of when to stop excising infected tissue. To excise more tissue will cause a larger wound and may result in greater deformity. Leaving dead infected tissue will almost certainly result in failure of healing. My experience has taught me that it is a much more common mistake to remove too little tissue than to remove too much. The less radical approach is justified on the grounds that, if the major focus of infection is drained and/or excised the local defence mechanisms will deal with residual areas. This view, although justified in principle, may produce an unsatisfactory result because the local defences are inefficient and the area of damaged tissue is frequently greater than expected. This applies particularly to infection in the plantar fat. An area of necrosis often occurs at the edge of a plantar incision. This is potentially dangerous for two reasons. First, there is uncertainty about the depth and extent of the necrosis. Second, the necrosis may spread beneath healthy skin until ultimately the viability of the skin is threatened. It will then be necessary to excise several square centimetres of skin in order to excise all the infected fat. Loss of this tissue can be prevented if a more aggressive approach to the removal of dead fat is adopted. If the infection is allowed to spread and involve the heel pad, it is unlikely that the foot will be saved.

Ischaemia

Ischaemic rest pain

The characteristics of this have been described on page 134. If this symptom is present it means there is an occlusion of the large blood vessels in the limb above the ankle. If arterial reconstruction is not feasible because of the general condition of the patient, the extent of the gangrene or, most commonly, the anatomy of the arterial obstruction, major amputation (see p. 182) is the likely outcome. The same result is likely following failure of a reconstruction.

Gangrene without rest pain

Absence of rest pain does not mean absence of arterial disease because neuropathy may keep even a severely ischaemic foot free from pain. Decisions may be very difficult to make with these patients and a plan of management based on detailed assessment of the circulation is shown in Fig. 9.13. Included in this group are patients with ulcers or gangrene, believed to be ischaemic in origin, which are not responding to adequate conservative measures.

Many elderly and/or frail patients with areas of gangrene can be managed conservatively without operation. The area of gangrene may be a single gangrenous toe or a necrotic slough covering a pressure area. If the gangrene is dry and localized and if the patient is free of ischaemic rest pain, conservative management may be continued. In many cases, the eschar or dead toe will separate and healing occur. Some patients die from other causes. The risk of this approach is that the blood supply will be inadequate and the consequent failure of healing will enhance the chances of developing spreading anaerobic sepsis. Infection serious enough to cause admission to hospital usually means abandoning the conservative approach, removing the dead tissue and ensuring adequate drainage. Failure of local surgery means that the patient must have a successful arterial reconstruction if the foot is to be saved (Fig. 10.3). The chances of successful reconstruction are unaltered by the previous local amputation although a greater loss of tissue is probable.

The alternative approach is to consider arterial surgery in all patients with significant ischaemia i.e. with absent ankle pulses. The most serious objection to this approach is that, even in the absence of ankle pulses, wounds and ulcers may heal if the collateral circulation is adequate and therefore arterial surgery is not needed. This successful result occurred in 89% of Sizer & Wheelock's (1972) series following local amputation. In these circumstances it is a serious error to submit the patient not only to angiography which is painful and carries small but definite risks of arterial occlusion or embolism, but also to the dangers and discomforts of a major operation (see p. 177 for an estimate of the risks of these operations).

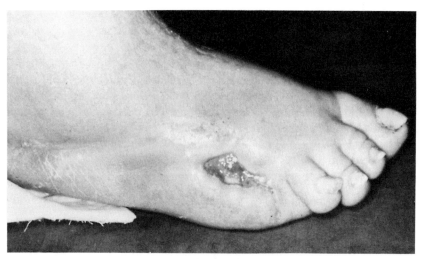

Fig. 10.3   Healing of foot following a successful femoropopliteal bypass. Previous amputation of the fifth toe had resulted in gangrene extending onto the dorsum of the foot.

Assessment of the adequacy of the circulation is critical and essential for optimal management (see p. 138). None of the tests is 100% accurate but intelligent use of them reduces, to an important degree, the uncertainty in the management of these patients.

Correction of deformity

Deformities of the feet that may predispose to the development of ulcers are common in diabetic patients. It is plausible to assert that surgical correction of these deformities would reduce morbidity by removing lesions that predispose to ulceration. However in Western communities, with a high prevalence of atherosclerosis, widespread adoption of this principle is hazardous. A variety of procedures may be performed ranging from correction of hallus valgus and hammer toes to the excision of prominent metatarsal heads (see p. 170). Textbooks of orthopaedic or podiatric surgery should be consulted for details of these procedures.

It is essential that the adequacy of the blood supply of the foot be determined before any elective surgery is performed on the foot of a diabetic patient. If the ankle pulses are impalpable the patient must be referred for detailed assessment of the circulation as outlined in Chapter 9. We still see several times each year patients in whom this advice has been ignored with disastrous results (see Fig. 10.4).

Neuropathic ulcers

Details of the treatment have been given on page 103. This may be con-

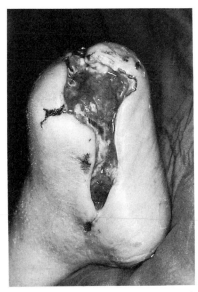

Fig. 10.4 Result of performing elective surgery for hammer toe in an ischaemic foot. Extensive necrosis and infection was controlled by femoropopliteal bypass and excision of dead tissue. The final result was good but there was a high price to pay for 'cosmetic' surgery.

tinued as long as there are no signs of deep abscess or osteomyelitis. In many patients the regimen can be continued for months or years, and may be repeated if an ulcer recurs. Such a policy requires meticulous supervision and this is very time-consuming. In addition, there is always the risk of infection which might result in the loss of more tissue. If an ulcer fails to heal or recurs several times it may be decided to attempt a cure by means of surgery. However, this should not be regarded as the easy solution because:

1. The operation carries risks of infection and failure of healing
2. The period of reduced mobility in or out of hospital lasts 4–6 weeks
3. Careful follow up is still required to prevent further lesions.

NON-OPERATIVE TREATMENT

The principles involved in non-operative treatment are rest and antibiotic therapy (see p. 72). A number of methods have been advocated in an attempt to avoid major amputation in patients with severe ischaemia who are unsuitable for arterial surgery. These will be discussed briefly.

Rest

The aim of treatment is to avoid the mechanical factors which precipitated the episode and thus to allow healing to occur. Strict rest in hospital is not often used, largely for economic and social reasons. In immobile or bed-ridden patients great care must be taken to avoid new pressure areas developing, so both feet must be carefully protected. The achievement of this simple aim requires meticulous nursing. The heels and the malleoli are the most vulnerable areas. A cradle is usually placed in the bed to keep the bedclothes off the feet.

A number of methods are used for protecting the feet and some are more effective than others. Boots made of sheepskin or synthetic material with similar properties are probably the best. They have the advantage of being easily removed to allow inspection of the foot. They should be made to cover as much of the foot as possible and if they are fixed by a strap across the dorsum of the foot, care must be taken that the strap is not too tight because pressure lesions can develop there too. If these boots are not available, a bulky cotton wool dressing kept in place by a crepe bandage is probably the next best choice. The wool must be thick over the heels and malleoli and the bandage must not be too tight. This is an important part of the postoperative dressings (see p. 167). Devices that use slings attached to bedframes are not recommended. They make nursing care more difficult, reduce the patient's mobility in the bed and, worst of all, are very difficult to keep properly positioned.

If the patient is allowed to continue walking, an effort should be made to allow a period of rest during the day. The benefits can be explained to the patient in simple mechanical terms, e.g. if walking is reduced by 20% then this will similarly reduce the stresses that caused the ulcer.

Other measures for relieving stresses on the foot have been described in Chapter 7. These include care of toe nails (p. 98), removal of hyperker-atotic skin (p. 101) and provision of splints and footwear (p. 103). All these important measures must be continued whether the patient is managed as an outpatient or an inpatient.

Non-operative treatment of gangrene

Many patients with gangrene due to ischaemia are considered unsuitable for arterial surgery. There are three major groups.

1. Elderly patients with gangrenous patches on the foot (see page 114).

2. Patients who present with extensive gangrene so that no useful part of the foot can be saved. This includes about one quarter of all patients presenting with severe ischaemia.

3. Patients with rest pain in whom arterial disease is not amenable to reconstruction.

The first group is frequently managed conservatively, attempting to avoid further trauma and giving antibiotic therapy for infection. For the other groups the pathway indicated in Figure 10.2 leads to major amputation and this is the most frequent outcome. A number of methods have been used to try to avoid this result in the third group. The common aim is to improve oxygen delivery to the skin and thus permit healing to occur. Several of the methods have undergone adequate clinical trials but none has come into widespread use.

1. Reduction in blood viscosity by haemodilution is important in patients with polycythaemia or thrombocythaemia. Haemodilution produces an increase in cardiac output and peripheral vasodilatation, while maintaining oxygen delivery to the tissues. (Shah et al 1980). The observed reduction in blood viscosity has led to the suggestion that chronic haemodilution might improve peripheral blood flow and thus promote the healing of ischaemic areas (Rieger et al 1979).

2. The induction of moderate hypertension, e.g. by use of mineralocorticoid drugs, can produce an improvement in distal blood pressure and flow which can be of clinical benefit (Lassen et al 1968). The side effects, particularly fluid retention, are potentially serious for patients with impaired myocardial function but with careful supervision complications can be avoided.

3. The infusion of vasoactive substances has been reported many times with mixed success. Patients with severe ischaemia have been successfully treated using intra-arterial infusion of prostaglandins (Szczeklik et al 1979, Sethi et al 1980). In view of the lack of benefit obtained from vasodilator drugs, the benefits of this regimen may have resulted from inhibition of platelet activity produced by the drug. Solcoseryl is a protein-free extract of calf blood which has been demonstrated to facilitate healing of lesions in patients with advanced atherosclerosis. It has been shown to be effective in avoiding amputations in patients with severe ischaemia (Charlesworth et al 1975). Its mode of action is unknown but in experimental situations it has been shown to increase oxygen uptake by tissue and this may be the reason for the improvement seen.

It is considered that vasodilator drugs have no place in the management of these patients, with or without diabetes. There has never been satisfactory evidence of benefit from their use, and there are strong theoretical arguments against them: it can be shown that the small vessels in severely ischaemic areas are already dilated and the only possible effect of vasodilator drugs is to shunt blood away from the affected areas by dilating normal vascular beds.

4. Hyperbaric oxygen therapy, applied either locally or systemically, should increase the oxygen available to the peripheral tissues. There have been limited reports of its successful use in diabetic patients.

Items 1–4 above have described reports providing reasonable evidence that the method advocated spared the patient a major amputation. In achieving this the treatments have been of significant benefit. Despite this potential, these methods are not widely used. There are several reasons for this, including the need for intra-arterial infusion and the potential side effects. In addition there is the doubt about the duration of relief. Does the patient really gain if amputation is postponed for only 3 months? Despite these objections, the potential benefits are great and the search for better methods of treatment will continue.

SURGERY

Pre-operative management

Control diabetes.   Good control of the diabetes will not be attained until infection has been drained but ketosis must be corrected and hyperglycaemia should be reduced, usually by insulin injections.

Control infection.   Antibiotic therapy is essential for about 24–48 hours before draining an infected foot, except in the presence of spreading anaerobic infection when operation is needed within hours of diagnosis. Pre-operative antibiotic therapy decreases the surrounding cellulitis and may reduce the chances of spread of septicaemia. But if there is a deep abscess, indicated by swelling of the foot and separation of the toes, antibiotics are never sufficient treatment.

Local amputation

A wide variety of local amputations may be performed to preserve a useful foot. The extent of the operation is governed primarily by the extent and spread of the necrosis and infection, and only secondarily by consideration of the appearance of the foot. The use of eponyms to describe these procedures has been kept to a minimum in this account. This is because improvization and opportunism, rather than detailed knowledge of numerous procedures, are important attributes of the surgeon confronted with these difficult problems.

It has long been an axiom that the first amputation should be the last. While this certainly applies to major amputations, it is an underlying theme of this section that, in the absence of a perfect method for estimating the adequacy of the blood supply, one attempt at a local amputation is often justified. However, as soon as it becomes clear that healing will not occur (often at the time of the first change of the wound dressings), urgent steps should be taken to determine if arterial reconstruction is possible. If it is not, further delay in performing the major amputation only reduces the chances of rehabilitation. Repeated attempts at successively higher amputations of the foot are to be deprecated.

The principles governing local amputations are:

1. Exploration and excision must be thorough but gentle. Remaining tissues must never be handled by anything harder than the surgeon's fingers or coarser than a skin hook.

2. Never use a tourniquet.

3. Infected areas must be opened wide (Fig. 10.5). There is no place for small incisions of fluctuant areas and insertion of drain tubes through the foot. There is usually deep infection, e.g. in bone, which cannot be drained adequately without wide incision and excision of devitalized tissue. The apparent gains from small incisions are outweighed by the losses from persistently draining sinuses and re-exploration for recurrent infection. If the blood supply is adequate a large incision will heal just as well as a small one.

4. Excise all dead tissue. Leaving dead tissue causes uncertainty about the extent of the lesion and provides a focus for recurrent infection.

5. Protect the other foot at all times. It may be the only one the patient will have.

Ray amputation

This operation, which removes a toe and the distal half of a metatarsal shaft, is considered by many to be the most useful of the local amputations. It

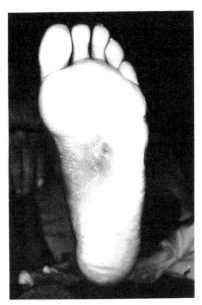

Fig. 10.5 Abscess pointing in sole of foot. An area of necrosis can just be seen at the base of the fifth toe. For adequate drainage the incision must extend from the base of the fifth toe, through the fluctuant area continuing for 2 cm or 3 cm towards the medial malleolus. Although the overlying skin appears healthy, there was extensive infection and necrosis beneath.

has the advantages of providing excellent drainage of the deep parts of the foot and removing the prominent metatarsal head beneath an ulcer. Posto-perative management, which is described in detail, can be applied to patients having the other operations discussed in this section.

Indications.   The operation is indicated for infection involving a single metatarsophalangeal joint arising from a trophic ulcer and for infection in the deep flexor tendon sheaths, e.g. arising from an infected gangrenous toe.

Technique.   It is essential that the operation provides adequate drainage of all infected areas of the foot. Collections of pus commonly form on the dorsum of the foot over the heads of the metatarsals. In the sole of the foot the infection tends to track medial to the heel pad, towards the tip of the medial malleolus.

The incision (Fig. 10.6a) encircles the base of the toe and extends proximally into the sole. It may pass through the ulcer, which need not be excised although minimal trimming of the thick skin in the area of the ulcer may be carried out. The toe is disarticulated at the metatarsophalangeal joint. The distal part of the plantar incision is deepened to the metatarsal shaft which is freed from its soft tissue attachment by dissection with a scalpel and a raspatory. The dorsal incision may be extended proximally if there is a collection of pus on the dorsum of the foot. This also facilitates mobilization of the metatarsal shaft. The bone is divided with bone cutters at approximately the middle of the shaft. Further proximal dissection is difficult and would damage the transverse arch.

This procedure results in a wound which, when viewed from the plantar aspect, is deepest distally and gradually becomes more superficial proximally (Fig. 10.6b, c). This allows blood and exudate to discharge onto the dressings and does not allow infected material to track proximally into the foot. The length of the incision is determined by the need to plan the wound

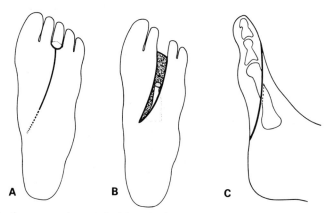

Fig. 10.6   Ray amputation. (a) Incision. (b) Appearance at end of operation. (c) Shelving appearance of wound seen from the side.

according to these requirements, and to drain the most proximal areas of infection. The skin wound should extend 1–2 cm proximal to the level of bone section. The wound is packed with gauze wet with a non-irritant solution, e.g. saline. The whole foot, including the heel, is then wrapped in a bulky cotton wool dressing, held in place by crepe bandages. The toes should be left exposed so they can be inspected and palpated.

Postoperative care. The principle of protecting the feet from further trauma must continue to guide management in the postoperative period. A cradle in the foot of the bed keeps the bedclothes clear and allows easy inspection. Narcotic analgesics are seldom needed because of the degree of neuropathy that is usually present. Severe pain is an urgent indication to inspect the wound. A 5 day course of antibiotic therapy should be completed. Fever should resolve within 36 hours of operation and any recrudescence is an indication to examine the wound. The wound should also be inspected if there is any suspicion of a deep infection in the leg, as suggested by fever, pain in the leg (not necessarily severe), and redness and swelling of the lower leg.

In the absence of any of these complications the dressings should be removed about the fifth postoperative day. This is best carried out in the operating theatre because there is often the need for further excision of small areas of necrotic tissue. If the facilities in the ward are adequate, the first dressing can be performed there and minor areas of necrosis may be excised. This careful revision of the wound is extremely important and may need to be repeated several times before the condition of the wound is satisfactory. Healing can occur despite small areas of necrosis but these provide foci from which recurrent abscesses may develop (Fig. 10.7). These often present several weeks after the patient has been discharged from hospital and, in addition to the inconvenience of repeating the whole process of drainage and review, there will be more loss of tissue.

Uncomplicated routines should be used for the subsequent management of these wounds. Dressings should be performed twice daily and comprise gauze soaked in saline or mild, non-irritant antiseptic. Astringents and enzymatic debriding agents should not be used. When the wound is free of necrotic tissue, it is sufficient to insert the edge of a gauze swab into the depths of the wound to keep the edges apart. This dressing can be changed daily in the ward until the wound is clean and granulating and then the edges can be allowed to fall together. There should be no hesitation in returning the patient to the operating theatre for further revision of the wound or excision of dead tissue should this be necessary. After about 14 days the bulk of the dressings may be reduced and the patient allowed to walk, with supervision, to the bathroom. A cautious approach should be adopted. The wound will take several weeks for complete healing but good cosmetic and functional results are likely.

This account of the operation and postoperative care has been given with what may seem to be obsessive attention to detail. No apology is made for

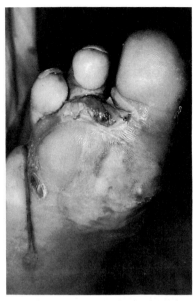

Fig. 10.7   Infection recurring after apparent satisfactory healing. The cause is failure to excise all dead and devitalized tissue.

this because failure to exercise sufficient care may result in loss of the foot and this should be regarded as great a disaster as, for example, the loss of a limb that has been operated on for intermittent claudication.

Toe amputations: single toe

Indications.   Amputation of a single toe is indicated either when there is gangrene of one digit in the absence of rest pain or when there is a perforating ulcer of the interphalangeal joint of the great toe.

Technique.   The technique varies with the digit involved. For the great toe the incision is made around the base of the toe and extended 2–3 cm proximally along the medial border of the foot. The tendons and soft tissues are divided and the toe disarticulated through the metatarsophalangeal joint. If there is any doubt about the cleanliness of the wound it should be left open for closure at a later date, but if the wound is apparently free of infection, the skin may be closed with adhesive paper tapes (e.g. Steristrips). Delay in closing the wound results in retraction of the skin flaps and closure may be impossible without removing part of the metatarsal head. However, if the wound is closed too early infection may result and this causes further loss of tissue. If there is adequate skin, it is not necessary to excise the head of the first metatarsal because preserving it leaves an important weight-bearing structure. If the degree of skin involvement means that the head of the first metatarsal cannot be preserved, the shaft of the bone should be divided obliquely to provide a rounded contour to the medial side of the foot.

Postoperatively, the patient need not as a routine be returned to the operating theatre for inspection of the wound. Walking may be allowed at about the end of the second week.

For the other toes it is usual to (1) incise the skin at the junction of living and dead tissue, (2) carefully strip the soft tissues from the bone, and (3) divide the bone through the base of the proximal phalanx or disarticulate at the metatarsophalangeal joint.

When carried out in this conventional manner the operation may fail because, when the patient is supine, the most dependent part of the wound into which exudate will drain has ready access to the deep tissues of the foot by way of the flexor tendon sheath which has been opened. These patients may present with a deep infection of the foot several weeks after apparently satisfactory healing. To avoid this complication the skin incision should be extended 1–2 cm proximally on either the plantar or dorsal aspect of the foot, so the wound can drain freely (see detailed description of ray amputation). This advice is contrary to the axiom that potentially ischaemic tissues are not incised. However in these patients infection not ischaemia is the greater problem. The wound should be managed as described for amputation of the great toe.

All (remaining) toes

The clawed toes on a neuropathic foot have a negligible role in walking but they are vulnerable to minor trauma and these episodes, if followed by infection, may cause major morbidity. If the blood supply of the foot is normal, amputation of healthy toes is sometimes justified. The patient is usually worried about the assault on his body image and will need (often along with his attending physician) reassurance that walking will be unaffected. It has been demonstrated that in normal subjects loads equivalent to about 30% of body weight are carried by the toes in the period just before the foot is lifted from the ground. In diabetics with neuropathy less than 10% of the body weight is borne by the toes during this phase of walking (see Ch. 6). This, combined with the observation of patients who have had all toes amputated (or even a transmetatarsal amputation), helps reassure the patient that his walking and balance will not be noticeably different from before operation.

Indications. This procedure can by carried out when there is repeated abrasion and ulceration of the dorsum of the toes that cannot be prevented by the provision of adequate footwear, and when there is a need to amputate (for other reasons) the great or fourth toe. Removal of the great toe makes the second toe particularly liable to trauma and subsequent removal of the second toe makes the remaining toes vulnerable successively. Removal of the fourth toe leaves a fifth toe which is both vulnerable and useless.

Technique. Incisions are made around the base of the toes and for a short distance down the medial and lateral sides of the foot (Fig. 10.8). The toes are disarticulated at the metatarsophalangeal joints and the wound closed with adhesive paper tapes. The final appearance is illustrated in Figure 10.9.

Excision of a metatarsal head

This procedure (Martin et al 1990) is based on the knowledge that increased load from a prominent metatarsal head is the cause of plantar ulceration (p. 88). It follows that removal of the prominent metatarsal head should allow healing of the ulcer.

Indication. This operation is indicated when plantar ulcer is either recurrent or persisting despite adequate conservative treatment. There must be no evidence of deep infections in the foot and the blood supply must be adequate.

Technique. A dorsal incision is made over the distal part of the appropriate metatarsal bone. The extensor tendons are displaced and the

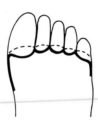

Fig. 10.8 Incisions for toe amputations. The medial and lateral extensions are necessary to allow dissection of the bases of the phalanges without vigorous retraction of the flaps.

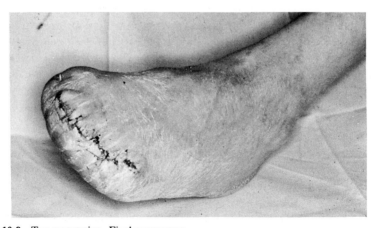

Fig. 10.9 Toe amputation. Final appearance.

incision deepened to bone. The neck and head of the metatarsal are separated by sharp dissection from their attachment and the metatarsophalangeal joint entered. The neck of the metatarsal is divided with bone cutters and the bone removed. The remaining tissues are allowed to fall together and the skin is closed with interrupted sutures. Prophylactic antibiotic therapy is continued for 5 days. The ulcer itself is not touched except for removal of hyperkeratotic skin.

Results.   Delbridge et al have reported primary healing in all their patients. This is a tribute to their procedures for selecting cases. However, ulceration recurred in 21%, illustrating the problems of removing a weight-bearing bone.

Transmetatarsal amputation

This is the classic local amputation for diabetics. The technique and results have been reported extensively by McKittrick et al (1949), and more recently by Wheelock (1961).

Indications.   This operation can be performed when there is gangrene involving more than one toe, and for persistent or recurrent plantar ulcer (Fig. 10.10).

At the present time we would use our laboratory tests (p. 151) to estimate the probability of healing and use this as an important factor in determining whether to perform a transmetatarsal amputation. In the absence of these tests, the conditions for the successful performance of the operation have been stated by Wheelock (1961) to be:

1. Gangrene must be localized to the toes and must not extend to the foot

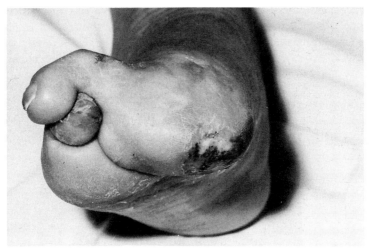

Fig. 10.10   Indications for transmetatarsal amputation. This patient has an ulcer over the first metatarsal head, a previous ray amputation and useless toes.

2. Infection must be localized
3. There must be no rest pain
4. Venous filling time must be not greater than 20 seconds
5. Dependent rubor must be absent or minimal.

Technique.   The incision across the dorsum of the foot is at the level of the middle of the metatarsal (Fig. 10.11). The plantar incision is at the base of the toes. These two incisions are joined along the medial and lateral borders of the foot. The plantar flap is dissected to contain as much soft tissue as possible and the dorsal incision is carried down to bone. The metatarsals are divided at the level of the dorsal incision. This can be carried out by an amputation saw, taking great care not to damage the skin flaps. Alternatively, the bones can be divided individually by a Gigli saw or bone cutters (the latter method may splinter the bones). Visible tendons are removed from the plantar flap which is then folded to approximate the dorsal incision. The wound is closed with adhesive paper tapes and produces a dorsally placed scar.

Discussion.   The surgeon must often choose between a ray and a transmetatarsal amputation. The former is preferred if there is a deep abscess in the foot because it provides better drainage. The ray amputation has the disadvantage that it reduces the number of weight-bearing metatarsal heads from five to four, while the transmetatarsal amputation preserves five metatarsals and may produce a better load distribution. However shortening the foot may produce greater stresses as discussed on page 80. Choosing between the two operations is most difficult with a patient referred for persistent or recurrent plantar ulceration. If a single ray is involved, we prefer to perform a ray amputation. Some prefer a transmetatarsal amputation if the first ray is involved, because of the belief that due to the high load carried by the first metatarsal there will be an unacceptable risk of recurrence if this bone is removed. My own view is that neither the clinical results nor the evidence from the studies of the mechanics of the foot strongly support this view. If two rays are involved, a transmetatarsal amputation is preferred

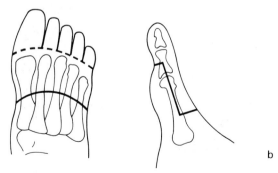

a   b

Fig. 10.11   Transmetatarsal amputation. (a) Dorsal view of incisions. (b) Medial view of incisions.

because of a high risk of recurrence if only three weight-bearing metatarsals remain (see Fig. 6.7). The indications and technique described by Wheelock have produced excellent results, but this may have been at the price of excluding from consideration many patients who had more extensive disease. It is conceded that broadening the indications will result in the inclusion of patients in whom a higher failure rate is to be expected and this will tend to discredit the procedure. However denying this procedure to these patients will result in the loss of many feet, when in many cases useful parts could be saved. It is in situations like this that difficult decisions arise. In general, if ischaemic rest pain is absent, it is reasonable to attempt a local amputation, and a variety of these 'ad hoc' procedures can be performed. The two major determinants of success are the care with which the operation is performed and the adequacy of the blood supply. Two specific examples will be discussed.

If infection or ulceration involves two rays, transmetatarsal amputation is preferred to ray amputation. The presence of infection deep in the foot is, conventionally, a contraindication to transmetatarsal amputation. However in these circumstances, transmetatarsal amputation with delayed closure of the wound and appropriate extension of the incisions to permit adequate drainage is an acceptable procedure (Fig. 10.12).

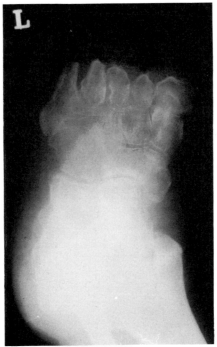

Fig. 10.12 Radiograph of foot after transmetatarsal amputation performed for extensive infection and necrosis. Healing occurred because the blood supply was good. The degree of shortening of the metatarsals is seen.

An important group of patients who may be helped by these operations are those who present with gangrene of the foot and in whom a successful arterial reconstruction has been performed. Conventional transmetatarsal amputation may be contraindicated because the necrosis often extends beyond the toes. In these cases, amputations may be performed more proximally in the foot, e.g. by disarticulating metatarsal from tarsal bones. As much plantar skin as possible should be preserved. Infected wounds should be left open and defects may be closed secondarily, sometimes by split skin grafts. By rigid application of the principles outlined and by meticulous wound care, many gratifying results can be obtained (Figs. 10.13, 10.14).

It can be argued that a formal Syme's amputation could be preferable in these circumstances. This may have the advantage of more rapid healing due to successful direct closure of the wound but preservation of the tarsal bones allows a normal shoe to be worn. This is a considerable long-term advantage which should not be discarded lightly.

Syme's amputation

For the reasons given above, I prefer to perform an amputation which preserves as much of the tissues of the foot as possible. However, some

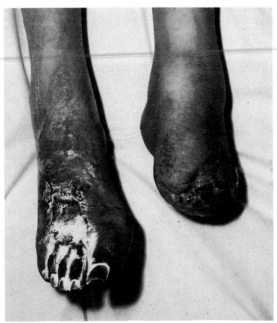

Fig. 10.13 The left foot shows the result obtained following femoropopliteal bypass, local amputation and skin graft for gangrene of the toes. An almost identical lesion developed in the right foot 12 months afterwards.

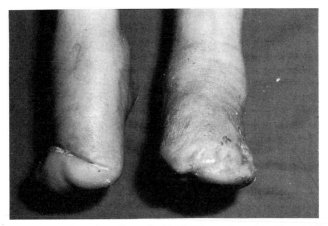

Fig. 10.14   Final result in patient shown in 10.13. The patient was able to walk without special footwear.

surgeons argue that the durability of the stump and the rapidity of healing still gives Syme's amputation a useful place. In these circumstances, the operation is indicated in a foot with gangrene that is too extensive to allow the safe performance of a transmetatarsal amputation, and in which the blood supply is judged to be sufficient to allow healing.

Technique.   The plantar incision is made from the tip of the lateral malleolus to a point 2 cm below the tip of the medial malleolus. The dorsal incision joins the ends of the plantar incision and divides the structures that run anterior to the ankle joint. On the medial side, the flexor tendons and plantar vessels and nerves are divided laterally, the peroneal tendons are encountered and divided. The ankle joint is entered by dividing its anterior ligament and the collateral ligaments are cut. These manoeuvres allow progressive plantar flexion of the foot. The posterior ligament is divided from within the ankle joint and the calcaneum is dissected from the heel flap. During this part of the procedure, great care must be taken to protect the branches of the posterior tibial artery which are closely applied to the posterior ligament, because the viability of the flap depends on their preservation. The malleoli are sectioned at, or just above the level of the ankle joint, ensuring that the cut is perpendicular to the long axis of the bones. The heel flap is brought forward and sutured in position.

The operation results in shortening of the limb by about 5 cm. The length and bulbous end of the stump make it difficult to fit a foot prosthesis. Some form of 'elephant-boot' appliance may give satisfactory functional results, and there are other prostheses designed to accommodate this stump.

THE DIABETIC AND ARTERIAL SURGERY

The whole range of procedures that may be performed on non-diabetics can be carried out successfully on diabetics. For detailed accounts of the procedures and the techniques for their performance, a textbook on arterial surgery should be consulted. This section is concerned with arterial surgery for disease affecting the leg in diabetics.

One of the major problems in the management of diabetic patients is to assess the role of arterial surgery. There are two major difficulties in this area. The first is the view that diabetics fare poorly after arterial surgery so arterial reconstruction is frequently not considered. However there are many reports which indicate that the results of arterial surgery on diabetics are only marginally inferior to the results obtained in non diabetics. As outlined in Chapter 3, the characteristic pattern of arterial disease in a diabetic is a relative sparing of the aorta and iliac arteries and an increase in atherosclerotic occlusions in the arteries of the calf. Severe disease of the calf vessels may preclude reconstructive surgery and the recognition of this pattern led to the view that diabetic patients were unsuitable for arterial reconstruction. It is true that arterial surgery cannot be performed in some diabetic patients, but this also applies to non-diabetics, although the number of patients considered inoperable is decreasing with the application of distal bypass surgery. The second major problem is the failure to recognize that, in a diabetic, gangrene may be treatable by local surgery without arterial reconstruction even if the axial arteries are obstructed. This has been discussed earlier in this chapter (p. 159).

Indications for arterial surgery

These are the same in the diabetic as in the non-diabetic limb, i.e. intermittent claudication, or threatened loss of limb.

Intermittent claudication

The diabetic patient with intermittent claudication should be considered for reconstruction according to the same criteria applied to the non-diabetic. If the claudication is severe enough to endanger employment or seriously interfere with domestic or leisure activities and the patient is unable to live within the limitations imposed by the claudication then surgery should be considered. The pain should have been stable for at least 3 months, or worsening. This delay is because there is a tendency for claudication of recent onset to improve as collateral vessels enlarge with the result that, after the concern at the initial development of the pain, the patient becomes able to live with the symptoms by adjusting his daily routines. The ability to walk no further than 100 metres may be a severe disability to one patient but may be easily tolerated by another of more sedentary habit. Another step which should be taken is to urge the patient to stop smoking. This may have two important effects. First, the progress of the vascular degeneration may be slowed and second, there is clear evidence that the chances of an arterial reconstruction remaining patent are higher if the patient has stopped smoking (Myers et al 1978).

The decision to offer an operation is also influenced by knowledge of the natural history of the disease, treated or untreated. The patient must be reasssured that the symptom of claudication does not carry a high risk of eventual loss of limb and this knowledge often markedly increases the patient's capacity to tolerate the pain. The attendants must also remember that there is a high (approximately 25%) risk that the patient will die of vascular disease in other areas, e.g. brain, heart or kidneys, within 5 years. The likely results of operation also influence the decision. Aortoiliac surgery when successfully performed has a good (about 80%) long-term patency. However, there is a significant mortality (1–5%) and this should be remembered before offering the patient an operation for a condition which does not directly threaten life. Femoropopliteal bypass surgery is safer (operative mortality about 1%) but is less effective in the long term. Many reports now suggest that about 50–60% of grafts are patent 5 years after operation. These results are leading many surgeons to the view that femoropopliteal bypass should be only infrequently performed for intermittent claudication. The conservative view is that operation for claudication should be delayed as long as possible because, in the event of failure of the bypass, the patient may be worse off and there may be only a slim chance of restoring the situation if the saphenous vein has been used already. The more aggressive approach is that the patient should be given the opportunity to enjoy what is left of a limited life expectancy. Whichever view is taken it must be remembered that a successful reconstruction is not the end of the patient's problems.

Once the decision has been made to consider surgery then, and only then, should angiography be performed. It should not be ordered until it has been decided that arterial surgery will be performed if the anatomy is favourable.

Threatened loss of limb

The conservative approach outlined above is not suitable when the survival of the limb is threatened. These patients need a major amputation unless the arterial supply to the foot can be improved. The clearest indication for action is ischaemic rest pain in the foot. Gangrene may or may not be present. These patients should be considered in the same way as non-diabetics. Arteriography should be performed to determine if arterial reconstruction is feasible. If reconstruction is not possible lumbar sympathectomy (p. 182) may be considered in an attempt to delay the need for amputation, although this is only worthwhile if the skin is intact. More difficult decisions arise in patients with coexisting neuropathy. These patients often have gangrenous patches over the heels and other pressure areas, or non-healing ulcers which are painless. Many of the patients are elderly and frail and in the absence of pain or spreading infection, no treatment is necessary.

A common and important group of patients comprises those with painless ulceration or gangrene which is not healing with conservative treatment and where there is evidence of impairment of the blood supply to the foot. It is assumed that any infection has been adequately drained. In these patients a local amputation may be considered despite serious doubts about the adequacy of the blood supply to the foot. If rest pain is present angiography should be performed with a view to carrying out an arterial reconstruction, preferably at the same time as the amputation. In the absence of rest pain and in the absence of any simple test which will allow the outcome to be predicted with confidence (see Ch. 9), the course most often chosen is to perform the local amputation. If it becomes apparent when the wound is inspected postoperatively that healing will not occur, angiography and successful reconstruction will be necessary if part of the foot is to be preserved.

Types of operations

The surgery carried out depends on the extent of arterial occlusion demonstrated on the arteriogram. The criteria are that there must be an adequate pressure above the area to be reconstructed and there must be patent vessels distal to the reconstruction so that the increased blood flow can be distributed to the peripheral tissues. This latter condition may not be satisfied if there is extensive occlusion of the arteries of the calf.

Aortoiliac stenosis or occlusion

To fulfil the first criterion given above, namely that there must be an adequate flow of blood into the reconstructed segment, aortoiliac stenosis or occlusion must be corrected before femoral artery occlusion is treated. The two techniques commonly used are insertion of a bypass graft (usually made of Dacron) from the aorta to each femoral artery (aorto-femoral bypass) or local disobliteration of the areas of narrowing or occlusion (thrombo-endarterectomy). The choice of operation depends on the experience of the surgeon and the extent of the disease, bypass being preferred if there is extensive disease and endarterectomy if the disease appears more localized, e.g. to one common iliac artery. Disease localized to the external iliac artery is particularly favourable to endarterectomy.

Surgery involving the abdominal aorta is dangerous. Any technical error is likely to require the transfusion of at least 1 litre of blood and, clamping the aorta causes a temporary impairment of renal and coronary function. To this must be added the cardiopulmonary effects of a major operation. For these reasons alternative approaches to the management of aortoiliac stenosis and occlusion have been developed. Two major options are available. If the disease is confined to one iliac system, a graft may be inserted from the femoral artery on the less affected side to the opposite femoral artery. This operation, femorofemoral crossover or bypass, carries a low risk and has a good long-term patency. The graft, which may be either vein or synthetic material, is commonly placed in the subcutaneous tissue across the pubis and its patency can be checked easily. It is often used in frail patients because of its safety. The alternative approach is to use the axillary artery as the donor vessel and connect it with the femoral artery via a long tube of Dacron or PTFE which is placed subcutaneously over the lateral thoracic wall. This operation, axillofemoral bypass, is also safe but has the disadvantage that use of a long prosthesis increases the chances of infection and occlusion. It is a reasonable alternative in patients unfit for aortofemoral bypass. If the iliac arteries are stenosed but patent, balloon angioplasty is the preferred treatment. This involves placing a catheter which includes a balloon across the stenosed segment. The balloon is inflated once it is in place across the stenosis. This disrupts the atheroma and produces an enlarged lumen. Operation is preferred if the artery is occluded or if the stenosis is long.

Femoral artery occlusion

The commonest lesion affecting the blood supply to the leg is an atherosclerotic occlusion near the point where the femoral artery passes through the hiatus in the adductor magnus muscle close to the shaft of the femur. Occlusion at this site commonly results in thrombosis of the femoral artery up to the next major branch — the profunda femoris artery. Some propagation of the thrombus occurs distally but the popliteal artery usually remains patent because of the flow around the knee through the collateral vessels which enter the popliteal artery. Stenosis of the profunda femoris artery is present in 20–30% of patients with femoral artery obstruction. The profunda femoris artery supplies the thigh muscles. Its terminal branches anastomose with the branches of the popliteal artery around the knee joint. The system of anastomoses may be so good that the patient is unaware of a femoral artery obstruction. Atheroma affecting the profunda femoris artery often involves only the first 1–2 cm and removal of this stenosing atheromatous material (profundaplasty) can improve the blood supply to the limb so that more distal reconstruction is unnecessary. This procedure has the further advantage that it requires only a groin incision and can, if necessary, be performed using local analgesia. The commonest procedure used to bypass obstruction of the femoral artery is a saphenous vein graft from the femoral artery above, to the popliteal artery below (femoropopliteal bypass). If the long saphenous vein is not available and the limb will be lost if reconstruction cannot be performed, there are a number of alternative procedures including the use of a synthetic tube but these grafts do not remain patent for as long as vein grafts.

In patients with symptoms of intermittent claudication, extensive disease of the calf vessels is regarded as a contraindication to operation. This is because the high fixed resistance of the distal arterial lesions limits blood flow through the graft and predisposes to occlusion. In patients in whom the survival of the limb is threatened, a less favourable situation may be accepted. Figure 10.15 shows the operative arteriogram obtained at the completion of a femoropopliteal bypass. There is no major vessel connected to the patent popliteal artery. Despite this severe disease, the operation was followed by healing of a foot ulcer and the graft was still patent when the patient returned for treatment of a similar lesion on the opposite side 3 years later (see Fig. 10.16). Femoropopliteal bypass may be attempted if there is a 3 cm or longer segment of popliteal artery patent and if a major amputation is the alternative. Frequently there is no usable popliteal artery

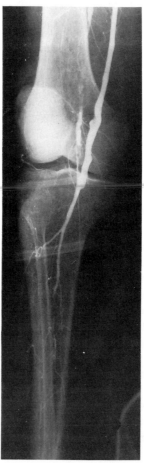

Fig. 10.15 Operative arteriogram at completion of a femoropopliteal bypass graft in a patient with severe disease of the calf arteries.

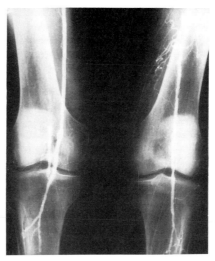

Fig. 10.16   Angiogram from same patient as Fig. 10.15 when she returned 3 years later (aged 76 years) for treatment of the opposite leg. The bypass remains patent.

and a bypass to one of the tibial vessels is the only possible procedure. Femoropopliteal bypass has a similar prognosis in diabetics and non-diabetics (Barner et al 1974, Cutler et al 1976, Rutherford et al 1988).

Femorocrural reconstruction

In recent years techniques have been developed to allow bypass grafting as far distally as the foot. These procedures, which should be performed only if the viability of the limb is threatened, can be carried out with reasonable success and may last for periods of several years. Functionally there are three terminal branches of the popliteal artery: the anterior tibial, posterior tibial and peroneal arteries. The peroneal artery ends on the lateral and posterior surface of the calcaneum but its perforating branch, which pierces the interosseus membrane 5 cm above the ankle joint and ends on the dorsum of the foot, may occasionally take the place of the dorsalis pedis artery. Any one of the three terminal branches of the popliteal artery may carry enough blood to allow the foot to survive and may be the only possible site for insertion of a bypass graft if the popliteal artery is occluded. The principles of these operations are similar to those for standard femoro-popliteal bypass but magnification is commonly used when carrying out the lower anastomosis. These operations can result in initial limb salvage in about half the patients (Reichle et al 1979). The initial success was less in diabetics (46% compared with 61% in non-diabetics), but the long-term results were similar in both groups. More recently Hurley et al (1987) have reported more favourable results in diabetics.

Lumbar sympathectomy

Removal of the lower part of the lumbar sympathetic chain removes the vasoconstrictor fibres to the skin of the foot. Within 24 hours of operation the foot becomes warm and dry: findings which give satisfaction to both surgeon and patient. However, close investigation suggests that these benefits are at best transient and at worst illusory. The blood flow to the foot is about five fold shortly after sympathectomy but this increase is not maintained, and after 2–3 weeks blood flow is about twice its preoperative value. There is no doubt, however, that many patients improve symptomatically following operation, but it is usually not possible to tell if this benefit is the result of operation or of the natural tendency to develop collateral pathways. In addition, it can be demonstrated that most of the increased blood flow is through channels that act as arteriovenous anastomoses. These vessels bypass the capillary network so that the blood flowing through them is of no nutritional value to the tissue.

Another argument is the one used against the exhibition of vasodilator drugs. The vessels in a severely ischaemic area are already dilated, presumably under the influence of local metabolites which are the most potent stimuli of local vasodilatation. Under these circumstances, removal of vasoconstrictor tone is likely to have the effect of lowering the resistance to flow through relatively normal vascular beds. This will shunt blood away from the ischaemic areas: an effect opposite to that which is desired. In diabetic subjects there is an additional argument against sympathectomy because the effects of the neuropathy may have been to produce degeneration of the sympathetic fibres. It can be argued that sympathectomy should only be considered in diabetics if vasoconstrictor tone can be demonstrated.

Despite these objections, lumbar sympathectomy may be of benefit to patients with ischaemic rest pain who have too much calf vessel disease to allow reconstruction, and in whom the skin of the foot is intact. If the ankle PI (see p. 140) is less than 0.25 the operation is futile. If ulcers or gangrene are present the chances of a clinically successful result are much reduced. Lumbar sympathectomy is less effective in diabetics than in non-diabetic patients as a means of avoiding amputation (DaValle et al 1981).

In performing the operation the aim is to denervate the vessels of the foot. This can be achieved by removing the fourth lumbar ganglion and short lengths of the adjacent sympathetic chain. It is no longer considered necessary to perform an extensive removal of the sympathetic chain between the renal and iliac vessels.

MAJOR AMPUTATIONS

The aim of the measures discussed in the preceding sections of this book has been to preserve the leg and avoid major amputation. However in many patients the state of the limb makes no other course feasible. Even at this stage it is important to maintain a hopeful outlook. Although the overall results of amputation are not good, there are few more grateful patients than those relieved of the constant pain of an ischaemic limb. The techniques of these operations and rehabilitation postoperatively do not differ in diabetics and non-diabetics and the reader is referred to other works (e.g. Little 1975) for details.

Below-the-knee amputation (BKA)

This is the operation of choice if major amputation is required. There is a good chance that the previously mobile patient will walk again if healing is successful. The patient can be provided with a modern prosthesis, held in place by only a strap around the knee, giving the least possible inconvenience to the patient. Use of this prosthesis requires less energy expenditure than needed with higher amputations. The disadvantage of the procedure is that with the incision more distally placed in the limb healing is less certain and most series have shown that the healing of a BKA is about 10% poorer than for higher amputations.

The need to undergo a major reamputation is very serious for the patient. The mortality is around 20% and there are the deleterious effects of a prolonged stay in hospital.

If major amputation is necessary, most surgeons will try to perform a BKA in a previously mobile patient. The techniques to predict healing of amputations have been described in Chapter 9, and their wider use might improve the results. Patients who are bedridden or whose mobility is limited by frailty present different problems. In these patients the greater certainty of healing of a higher amputation is usually accepted. The major requirement of the limb is then to provide stability when seated and the ability to turn over in bed and these aims can be achieved by an amputation performed at or just above the knee joint. There is a further disadvantage of a BKA in these patients. Flexor contracture of the knee joint is likely to occur and this provides another deformity to be coped with by the attendants. In these patients the BKA offers no advantages to counter the disadvantages described.

Preoperative preparation

Once the decision to recommend major amputation has been made, the consent of the patient must be obtained. In many cases the patient realizes that the limb is useless but in others, particularly when there has not been severe pain, the idea of an amputation comes as a shock. The person counselling the patient should gently explain that the foot is both useless and a threat. The level of amputation should be indicated and the stages of the procedure explained. It should be pointed out that a patient who was mobile before the condition of the limb deteriorated can expect to be rehabilitated. The patient should be warned of the possibility of phantom pain and reassured that this sensation will be temporary. The help of the physiotherapist should be enlisted to explain the need for quadriceps exercises and to instruct the patient in their performance.

Technique

A variety of techniques is available; that using a long posterior musculocutaneous flap will be described. This is favoured because of empirical observations, later supported by skin blood pressure studies, that the pretibial skin has a worse blood supply than the skin over the back of the calf. As a result ischaemic necrosis of the skin occurs most often at the distal edge of the anterior flap.

The skin incisions are marked out. The anterior incision is horizontally placed 10 cm below the tibial tuberosity and extends from the fibula laterally, halfway around the limb. From the ends of this mark, lines are drawn 10–12 cm distally in the long axis of the limb and the distal limits of these marks are joined transversely.

Much of the operation is carried out from the front of the limb. The anterior incision is carried through superficial and deep fascia. The anterior crural muscles are divided and the anterior tibial vessels, which lie close to the interosseus membrane, are divided and ligated. The muscles surrounding the fibula are divided and the fibula cut with a Gigli saw 1 cm proximal to the intended line of section of the tibia. The posterior flap is now raised. At its distal limit it will divide the proximal part of the tendo calcaneus, and more proximally it includes the gastrocnemius muscle. The next step is the division of the tibia. The periosteum is elevated 1 cm proximal to the intended line of section and a bevel is cut at 45° through the anterior 1 cm of the tibia. Note that this is the only dissection performed beneath the anterior flap. The division of the tibia is completed by a transverse saw cut. The lower leg and foot are now attached only by the deep posterior muscles of the calf. These are divided with a scalpel or amputation knife and the limb is removed. Bleeding from the cut ends of venous sinuses in the gastrocnemius muscle is usually more prominent than bleeding from the posterior tibial and peroneal vessels. Haemostasis is secured by clamping and ligating bleeding vessels. The posterior flap is now folded forwards over the tibia and its alignment inspected. It may be shortened if it has been cut too long. Dense collagenous tissue (tendon), which has a poor blood supply, may be excised from the distal part of the flap. If too much of the gastrocnemius muscle bulk has been retained, part of it may be excised but the amount removed should be the minimum necessary to allow the posterior flap to be approximated without tension to the anterior flap. The deep fascia of the flaps may be sutured with chromic catgut or polyglycolate sutures and the skin is closed with fine interrupted silk or nylon sutures or, preferably, with adhesive paper tapes.

The difference in the lengths of the perimeter of the flaps often results in small 'dog ears' at each end. On no account should they be trimmed because this involves incisions into the flaps and impairs their blood supply. Remodelling of the wound makes the 'dog ears' inconspicuous by the time the prosthesis is fitted. Haemostatis should be good enough to make a drain tube unnecessary. The wound is covered with gauze and the stump wrapped in a bulky dressing of cotton wool held in place by crepe bandages.

Postoperative management

The patient may require occasional doses of narcotic analgesics but severe pain is an urgent indication for inspection of the wound. Cellulitis surrounding the wound requires that a swab be taken and immediately examined for microorganisms, especially gram-positive bacilli. Phantom pain is very common but not often severe. If the patient experienced severe pain before operation, he often considers that the pain from the wound is much less than the pain from the ischaemic foot.

The most important part of the postoperative management is physiotherapy. From the first postoperative day the patient should perform quadriceps exercises under supervision. These must be continued energetically until the prosthesis is fitted. The quadriceps group of muscles is the major factor producing stability of the knee joint and the patient can be told that the length of time before he walks again is dependent to a large degree on the strength of these muscles. The dressings are left undisturbed for 7 days provided that pain, fever or discharge do not indicate the need for earlier inspection of the wound. A lighter dressing can then be applied and attention directed to careful bandaging to minimize oedema formation in the stump. Sutures, if used, should remain for 14–21 days.

Variations

Design of the flaps.   There are several possible alternative ways of designing the anterior flap. The flap may be made semicircular and 5–6 cm long. At the other extreme, surgeons who are very worried about necrosis in this area may excise anterior tibial skin for 1–2 cm above the proposed line of bone section (called a 'negative' anterior flap).

Guillotine amputations.   If the amputation is being performed in the presence of sepsis, the operation may be planned so that the wounds are left open. The classic guillotine amputation divides all tissues at one level. This has the major disadvantage that retraction of the skin causes a long delay in obtaining skin cover. A more practical alternative is the operation described by Silbert and advocated for use in diabetics by Catterall. In this operation, the skin and subcutaneous tissue are divided circumferentially at a level 5 cm below the site of bone section and folded back to permit division of the bones and remaining soft tissues. The skin flaps are then replaced and the cavity filled with Vaseline gauze. If the length of the flaps has been well judged, retraction of the skin flaps and healing will result in a soundly healed stump with a small stellate scar over its end. More recently Catterall (1978), who has extensive experience of the treatment of diabetics, has preferred the long posterior flap technique described earlier.

Complications

Necrosis. Death of the wound edges results in failure of healing and this is the most serious local complication of amputation. Infection may be a factor, but usually necrosis occurs because the local blood supply is inadequate to maintain the viability of the tissues. Tight sutures are an important cause and, although many experienced surgeons regularly suture amputation wounds, it is believed that the technique of wound closure using adhesive paper tapes is more likely to be 'fail-safe'. Necrosis of a few millimetres of the wound edge is compatible with successful healing, but if the greatest width of the necrotic area is greater than 1 cm, a long delay in healing will be the best result and higher amputation may be necessary. If substantial areas of necrosis are present, they should be excised at the junction of living and dead tissues and secondary healing awaited.

Persistent pain in the wound is a bad prognostic sign. A wound which has an adequate blood supply and is adequately immobilized becomes much less painful after a few days. Persistent pain which is not due to infection suggests that the blood supply is inadequate and the wound may fail to heal. Absence of pain, however, does not guarantee success. In a severely neuropathic and ischaemic limb a wound may fail to heal although pain has been minimal or absent. This sequence is more common following foot amputations than following BKA.

Infection. One of the important effects of prophylactic antibiotics has been the virtual elimination of gas gangrene in patients having major amputations. The proximity of the wound to a reservoir of organisms, i.e. the anus, and the resistance of sporing organisms to skin disinfectants, combined with the presence of relatively ischaemic muscle, creates the ideal conditions for the establishment of an anaerobic infection. Penicillin is the agent of choice and should be given with the premedication, and for 24 hours after operation (see p. 72).

Ischaemia as a cause of wound pain has already been mentioned. Infection is another important cause. In the most serious cases, when gas gangrene develops, there will be a thin exudate from the wound and rapidly spreading muscle tenderness in a seriously ill patient. If examination of a smear of the exudate reveals the presence of sporing organisms, then urgent treatment must be undertaken (see p. 123). Fortunately, this is now a very rare sequence of events. Mixed infection which may include staphylococci, anaerobic bacilli and intestinal gram-negative organisms are much more common. The presence of necrotic tissue is an important contributing factor to the establishment of these infections, and this is one of the reasons why meticulous operative technique is necessary. If pyogenic infection becomes established, it is treated using standard principles.

Haemorrhage. The formation of a haematoma in the wound delays healing and predisposes to infection. The best prevention is careful haemostasis in the wound — a drain tube does not compensate for untidy surgery. A haematoma should be evacuated by reopening a short length of the wound and re-bandaging the stump firmly. Remember that bandages which are too tight cause ischaemia. Secondary haemorrhage was once a feared complication following amputation. This probably occurred following the amputation of limbs with a good blood supply, e.g. following trauma or infection. In performing a BKA the major arteries may often be divided without major bleeding so that secondary haemorrhage is a very uncommon event.

Later complications. The amputation stump remains a vulnerable area. An apparently healed wound may be split open, usually following a fall, several weeks after operation. In addition, progression of ischaemia may result in ischaemic rest pain and ischaemic necrosis of the stump. Ulcers developing from excessive pressure from a poorly fitting prosthesis are another important cause of morbidity. If flexion contraction is allowed to develop it usually means that the patient will never manage a below knee prosthesis.

Serious difficulties occur in about 25% of patients (Little et al 1974).

Higher amputations

If a BKA is considered inapplicable, or if it fails to heal, a higher amputation may be necessary. The operation chosen will depend on the preference of the surgeon, the chances of fitting a prosthesis and the extent of the arterial disease. The three operations most commonly performed are a through-knee disarticulation, a supracondylar (Gritti-Stokes) amputation and a midthigh amputation. The first two owe their successful healing to the anatomy of the collateral arteries which, in the area of the knee joint, are in the subcutaneous tissue. In addition both operations involve the division of only small amounts of muscle tissue which has the practical advantage of making haemostasis easier and the theoretical advantage of decreasing the chances of anaerobic sepsis. Further, both operations preserve maximum length of limb to facilitate the management of a bed-ridden patient. The major disadvantages of the operations relate to the difficulties in fitting a prosthesis. The length of the stump means that the knee joint of a prosthesis must be placed lower than on the intact side. In addition, the bulbous lower end of the femur following a through-knee operation is more difficult to accommodate. Difficulty in fixing the patella following a supracondylar amputation may also cause problems for the prosthetist. Most patients in this group are not expected to walk again and in these cases I prefer to perform a through-knee or supracondylar amputation if a BKA is not feasible. If reamputation is needed following failure of a BKA, the proximity of the anterior skin incision to the area of ischaemia or necrosis usually means that a mid-thigh amputation is necessary.

REHABILITATION

There are two major aims when considering a patient for possible amputation:

1. To produce healing by removing a painful and/or infected and therefore dangerous limb or part of a limb
2. To restore mobility.

The achievement of the second aim begins preoperatively when the nature of the operation is discussed. While many patients would rather die than have a leg amputated, most respond to a positive attitude on the part of their advisors who should emphasize the relief of pain, the removal of a dangerous or useless limb and the chances of walking again. An approximate timetable for the fitting of the prosthesis may be given. This depends on local policies and the availability of limb-fitting facilities. In a patient having a BKA the importance of quadriceps function must be emphasized.

The greatest contribution to rehabilitation is made by the surgeon who carefully and meticulously performs the operation, because a major factor delaying rehabilitation is problems with the amputation wound.

It is following the operation that the widest divergence in practices occurs. The conventional conservative approach has been to await healing of the wound and then refer the patient to a specialist in limb-fitting and rehabilitation who undertakes the subsequent management, often at another centre. At the other extreme all amputations are performed by a single group of surgeons, immediate fitting of a prosthesis is undertaken, and a co-ordinated programme of aggressive rehabilitation is begun. The results which can be achieved by this type of programme are shown by the report of Malone et al (1979) when 50 per cent of below-knee amputees had a definitive prosthesis fitted within 32 days of operation. The only reservation held about these results is that they may have been a highly selected group of patients. However most surgeons would be pleased to achieve these results, even if they were able to select their patients!

A major difference between the two approaches is the immediate fitting of the prosthesis. This has the advantages that the wound is immobilized so that pain is less and healing is better, the stump does not become oedematous so that fitting a definitive prosthesis is easier and the patient can bear weight on the amputated limb within a few days of operation. These advantages may represent a considerable benefit for the patient. The reduction in pain and early mobility are good for morale and the maintenance of muscle power, and any resulting reduction in hospital stay is obviously beneficial. The disadvantage is that necrosis and infection may not be detected until late because of the unwillingness of attendants to remove the rigid dressing. This may result in serious problems for the patient should these complications occur. In addition, the best results are likely to be obtained if there is a team which is regularly using the technique and which has adequate resources to function efficiently.

An intermediate course is to use a prosthesis based on an air-filled splint as described by Little (1971). This device consists of a standard air splint supported by a metal socket with a prosthetic foot attached. In the early postoperative period the air splint provides support for the wound. Subsequently it provides the socket which joins the limb to a temporary prosthesis. This method has the great advantage that the air splint can be removed when necessary and reapplied easily.

There is a strong argument for forming a rehabilitation team to serve a large hospital or groups of hospitals. The evidence suggests that the money saved by such groups would pay the costs many times over and many more patients would be walking sooner.

PROGNOSIS

The outlook for diabetic patients with major foot lesions is not good. There are some young patients with insulin-dependent diabetes mellitus who develop neuropathic ulceration or infection and who, following treatment, live for many years without further treatment. However, for an elderly atherosclerotic diabetic patient, the development of gangrene of the foot may result in amputation and death within a short period of time. The overall results depend on the case mix. In our series (Faris et al 1988), in which the mean age of patients was 69 years, half the patients either died or lost the limb within two years of presenting for treatment (Fig. 10.17) (also Taylor & Porter 1987).

Diabetes is the most common cause of a major amputation of the lower limb. The risk in diabetics is about 15 times above that of the non-diabetic population (Most & Sinnock 1983). More than 50 000 amputations were performed on diabetic patients in the USA in 1985 (Bild et al 1989).

The outlook for patients having major amputations is poor; operative mortality is about 10% and more than half the diabetic patients will be dead in two years (Finch et al 1980). The prognosis for the remaining limb is not favourable. About half the surviving patients develop a new lesion within 2 years and some of these require amputation (Goldner 1960, Brodie 1970). The results of rehabilitation of surviving patients are also poor; only about half become independently mobile or mobile beyond their own homes. (Little et al 1974; Finch et al 1980).

These gloomy figures should not deter us from using our best endeavours to allow these patients to enjoy the remainder of their lives as comfortably

Overall survival

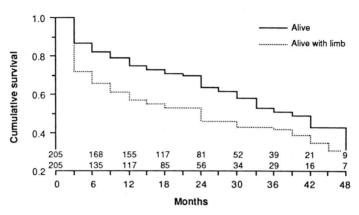

Fig. 10.17 Life table analysis showing survival with and without amputation. In 2 years, approximately half the patients have either died or undergone amputation. From Faris et al 1988.

as possible. Achieving this objective requires considerable effort and attention to detail, as has been emphasized repeatedly throughout this book. In spite of the inevitable disappointments many gratifying results can be obtained and this can be a source of considerable satisfaction to those involved.

REFERENCES

Barner H B, Kaminski D L, Codd J E, Kaiser G C, Willman V L 1974 Haemodynamics of autogenous femoropopliteal bypass. Archives of Surgery 109: 291–293

Bild D E, Selby J V, Sinnock P, Browner W S, Braveman P, Showstack J A 1989 Lower extremity amputation in people with diabetes — epidemiology and prevention. Diabetes Care 12: 24–31

Brodie I A O D 1970 Lower limb amputation. British Journal of Hospital Medicine 4: 596–604

Catterall R C F 1978. In: Oakley W G, Pyke D A, Taylor K W, Diabetes and its management, 3rd edn. Blackwell Scientific Publications p. 169

Charlesworth D, Harris P L, Palmer M K 1975 Intra-arterial infusion of Solcoseryl: a clinical trial of a method of treatment for pregangrene of the lower limb. British Journal of Surgery 62: 337–339

Cutler B S, Thompson J E, Kleinsasser L J, Hampel G J 1976 Autologous saphenous vein femoropopliteal bypass: analysis of 298 cases. Surgery 79: 325–331

DaValle M J, Baumann F G, Mintzer R, Riles T S, Imparato A M 1981 Limited success of lumbar sympathectomy in the prevention of ischemic limb loss in diabetic patients. Surgery Gynecology and Obstetrics 152: 784–788

Faris I B, Duncan H, Young C 1988 Factors affecting outcome of diabetic patients with foot ulcers or gangrene. Journal of Cardiovascular Surgery 29: 736–740

Finch D R A, MacDougall M, Tibbs D J, Morris P J 1980 Amputation for vascular disease: the experience of a peripheral vascular unit. British Journal of Surgery 67: 233–237

Goldner M G 1960 The fate of the second leg in the diabetic amputee. Diabetes 9: 100–103

Hurley J J, Auer A I, Hershey F B, Binnington H B, Woods J J, Nunnelee J D, Milyard

M K 1987 Distal limb reconstruction: patency and limb salvage in diabetics. Journal of Vascular Surgery 5: 796–800

Lassen N A, Larsen O A, Serensen A W S, Hallbook T, Dahn I, Nilsen R, Westling H 1968 Conservative treatment of gangrene using mineralocorticoid-induced moderate hypertension. Lancet 1: 606–609

Little J M 1971 A pneumatic weight-bearing temporary prosthesis for below-knee amputees. Lancet 1: 271–273

Little J M 1975 Major amputations for vascular disease. Churchill Livingstone, Edinburgh

Little J M, Petritsi-Jones D, Kerr C 1974 Vascular amputees: a study in disappointment. Lancet 1: 791–795

Martin J D, Delbridge L, Reeve T S, Clagett G P 1990 Radical treatment of mal perforans in diabetic patients with arterial insufficiency. Journal of Vascular Surgery 12: 264–268

McKittrick L S, McKittrick J B, Risley T S 1949 Transmetatarsal amputations for infection of gangrene in patients with diabetes mellitus. Annals of Surgery 130: 826–842

Malone J M, Moore W S, Goldstone J, Malone S J 1979 Therapeutic and economic impact of a modern amputation programme. Annals of Surgery 189: 798–802

Most R S, Sinnock P 1983 The epidemiology of lower extremity amputations in diabetic individuals. Diabetes Care 6: 87–91

Myers K A, King R B, Scott D F, Johnson N, Morris P J 1978 The effect of smoking on the late patency of arterial reconstruction in the legs. British Journal of Surgery 65: 267–271

Reichle F A, Rankin K P, Tyson R R, Finestone A J, Shuman C R 1979 Long-term result of femoroinfrapopliteal bypass in diabetic patients with severe ischaemia of the lower extremity. American Journal of Surgery 137: 653–656

Reiger H, Kohler M, Schoop W, Schmid-Schonbein H, Roth F J, Leybe A 1979 Haemodilution in patients with ischaemic skin ulcers. Klinische Wochenschrift 57: 1153–1161

Rutherford et al 1988 Factors affecting the patency of infrainguinal bypass. Journal of Vascular Surgery 8: 236–246

Sethi G K, Scott S M, Takaro T 1980 Effect of intra-arterial infusion of PGE in patients with severe ischaemia of lower extremity. Journal of Cardiovascular Surgery 21: 185–192

Shah D M, Prichard M N, Newell J C, Karmody A M, Scovill W A, Powers S R 1980 Increased cardiac output and oxygen transport after intraoperative isovolemic, hemodilution. Archives of Surgery 115: 697–700

Sizer J S, Wheelock F C 1972 Digital amputation in diabetic patients. Surgery 72: 980–989

Szczeklik A, Nizankowski R, Skawinski S, Szczeklik J, Gluszko P, Gryglewski R J 1979 Successful treatment of advanced arteriosclerosis obliterans with prostacyclin. Lancet 1: 1111–1114

Taylor L M, Porter J M 1987 The clinical course of diabetics who require feet surgery because of infection or ischaemia. Journal of Vascular Surgery 6: 454–9

Wheelock F C 1961 Transmetatarsal amputation and arterial surgery in diabetic patients. New England Journal of Medicine 264: 316–320

Index